A Manual of
Neuro-Anatomical Acupuncture

Volume I:
Musculo-Skeletal Disorders

Joseph Y. Wong, MD, FRCP(C), PhD, CAFCI

SCARBOROUGHS LTD
Acupuncture Suppliers
(01460) 72072

First Canadian Edition 1999

Copyright © 1999 The Toronto Pain and Stress Clinic Inc.

This book is distributed by:
Skill Developments Home & Overseas Ltd
56 Jervis Crescent
Birmingham UK B74 4PN
UK Tel: 44(0)121 353 1912
UK Fax: 44(0)121 353 0981

The copyright of this book is registered under The Canadian registration number: 475920.

No part of this book may be reproduced, stored in a retrieval system, or transmitted in any form or by any means, electronic, mechanical, photocopying, recording, or otherwise, without the prior written permission of the copyright owner.

ISBN 0-9685194-0-7

Printed in Canada

About the Author

Joseph Y. Wong, MD; FRCP(C); PhD; CAFCI

- Western medicine and acupuncture of more than 40 years experience
- Certified medical specialist in rehabilitation medicine
- Fellow of Royal College of Physicians, Canada
- Former specialist consultant in rehabilitation medicine: Toronto General Hospital, Toronto; Wellesley Hospital, Toronto; Lyndhurst Spinal Hospital, Toronto
- Former Department Head in Rehabilitation Medicine Department: St. Joseph Hospital, Toronto; Laurentian Hospital, Sudbury
- Chief Lecturer and Examiner, Acupuncture Foundation of Canada Institute, for 25 years
- Member of American Academy of Medical Acupuncture (Certified)
- Lecturing neuro-anatomical acupuncture in the world: Canada, USA, UK, New Zealand, China, Sri Lanka
- Recipient of Ph.D. (Honoris Causa), The Open International University for Complementary Medicines
- Author: Manual of TENS
  The Science of Acupuncture Therapy

Dedicated to Angi

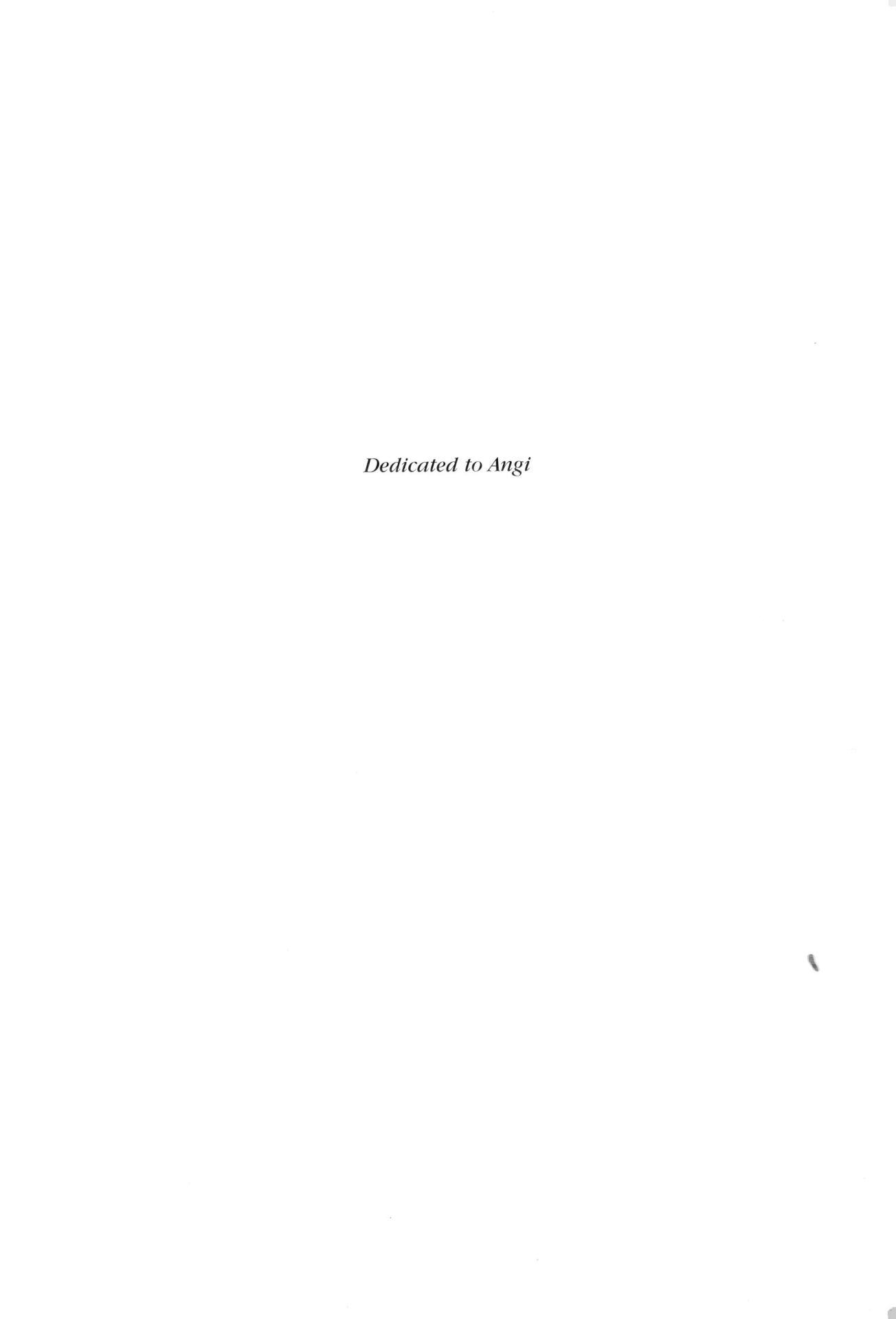

RAPIDS

Rivers run
Throughout history, time
and us.

Rivers damned, dammed, diverted.

Oxbows form,
and pebbles drop.

Ripples spreading out
in us, in time, in space.

Sorcery flows to science.

We portage,
or stagnant – camp,
or rejoice in the rapids.

This was old when time was young.

The pilots learned, the rocks to shun.

And down the course,
The rivers run.

CHARLIE SMITH

Acknowledgements

- My deepest gratitude to my wife, Marta Wong, for her devoted assistance and loving support.

- My sincere gratefulness to the artists and designer:
    Cynthia Dahl
    Ben Spergel
    Philip Sung

- My special thanks to the computer advisers:
    Anson Wong
    Ron Erwin

- My genuine appreciation to the English editor:
    Lee Danes

- My heartfelt admiration for the poet:
    Charlie Smith

Table of Contents

Page

Chapter One	Evolution of Acupuncture	1
Chapter Two	Summary of Traditional Chinese Medicine (TCM)	3
Chapter Three	Basic Meridians in Traditional Chinese Medicine	11
Chapter Four	Standard Acupuncture Nomenclature	17
Chapter Five	Acupuncture as a Physical Therapy	27
Chapter Six	The Biochemical Mechanism of Acupuncture	31
Chapter Seven	Acupuncture in Pain Management	39
Chapter Eight	The Acupuncture Treatment	45
Chapter Nine	Neuro-Anatomical Acupuncture	61
Chapter Ten	Normalization of the Autonomic Nervous Dysfunction with Acupuncture	67
Chapter Eleven	The Therapeutic Strategies of Neuro-Anatomical Acupuncture	73
Chapter Twelve	The Possible Hazards and Complications of Acupuncture	79
Chapter Thirteen	The Neck	85
Chapter Fourteen	The Back and the Perineum	111
Chapter Fifteen	The Shoulder	135
Chapter Sixteen	The Elbow and the Forearm	153
Chapter Seventeen	The Wrist and the Hand	173
Chapter Eighteen	The Hip	187
Chapter Nineteen	The Knee and the Leg	207
Chapter Twenty	The Ankle and the Foot	227

Introduction

The mechanism of acupuncture effect has been increasingly understood through scientific research in the world. It is my intention to put the East and West together for the enhancement of medical practice. With this in mind, I am writing a series of books on the basis of anatomy and physiology, especially for the medical and para-medical professionals who may find the TCM classical methodology not easily comprehensive.

This series of books has six volumes:

Volume I	Neuro-Anatomical Acupuncture for Musculo-Skeletal Disorders
Volume II	Neuro-Anatomical Acupuncture for Neurological Disorders
Volume III	East meets West, A Review of TCM with Western Medicine Interpretation
Volume IV	Neuro-Anatomical Acupuncture for Cardio-Vascular and Respiratory Disorders
Volume V	Neuro-Anatomical Acupuncture for Genito-Urinary and Gastro-Intestinal Disorders
Volume VI	Neuro-Anatomical Acupuncture for Stress and Mental Disorders

These books are in the format of a manual. My attempt is to have them presented with simplicity and clarity.

Joseph Wong

Chapter One

Evolution of Acupuncture

It is believed that acupuncture had already begun as early as the Stone Age. Significant advances in acupuncture were made in the Bronze and Iron Ages (407 - 310 BC.). The philosophical principles of yin and yang and the five elements were conceived in the Han Dynasty (206 BC - AD 220). During this time, the ancient healers developed the fundamental theories forming the basis of Traditional Chinese Medicine.

During the movement from dynasty to dynasty, more medical knowledge was gained and both the theory and practice of acupuncture were gradually becoming more systematically organized. Through the Yuan and Ming Dynasties (AD 907-1636), acupuncture was further advanced, becoming more sophisticated due to an extensive review and collection of formal clinical documents and literature.

In 1840, during the Ching Dynasty, Opium War broke out in China. This was followed by the revolution of China in 1911. Within this time, the main gate of China was opened to the Western world. As a result, Western medicine was introduced to China. At the same time, acupuncture began to be regarded as a medical superstition rather than a true medical science. Because of this, acupuncture suffered a great decline.

In the 1950's, under the Communist Party of China, acupuncture moved into a new era, as Traditional Chinese Medicine began to re-emerge and be integrated with Western medicine. As a matter of fact, prior to this time, acupuncture remained unchanged for at least two thousand years, both in terms of its basic theory and its clinical practice. This status could be due, at least in part, to a strong belief that tradition should be honored without challenge.

In the 1960's, Chinese medicine, including acupuncture, made transmission to the West and underwent further adaptation to the twentieth century, particularly after the discovery that acupuncture affected neurotransmitters.

Within the past twenty-five years, there has been a very rapid growth in scientific advances in acupuncture research throughout the world.

It is extremely intriguing to see this ancient medical art becoming a part of the development of highly modern world medical advances. I am a member of the American Academy of Medical Acupuncture. The Academy's certificate bears four Chinese letters, gu wai jin yung, 古為今用, meaning "Put the ancient to today's practice". Hopefully, we have learned that we must not discard ancient knowledge and practices. In fact, ancient heritages are like very rich treasure boxes and we should, therefore, continue to dig into them in order to find more valuables. However, we should study these valuables with our modern science, rather than just adopting them without careful examination and thorough comprehension. I strongly believe that the neuro-anatomical approach to acupuncture takes us in the right direction, both for the future of acupuncture and the advancement of medicine. The ongoing evolution of acupuncture is central to new and exciting changes in both Eastern and Western approaches in medicine to healing and prevention.

Chapter Two

Summary of Traditional Chinese Medicine (TCM)

Basic Characteristics of TCM

Holism

- unity and integration of the body and the relationship of the natural world to human beings

- human body and the external environment together as an organic whole

- universe: macrocosm
  human being: microcosm

- studying holistic relationship between macrocosm and microcosm

- studying physiology, pathology, diagnosis and treatment in human medicine

Treatment Based Upon Syndrome Differentiation

- using four diagnostic methods: inspection (i.e. tongue diagnosis), auscultation and olfaction, interrogation, palpation (i.e. pulse diagnosis)

- analysis of information to provide foundation for syndrome differentiation

- treatment based on syndrome differentiation

Yin/Yang and Five Elements

In TCM, the theories of yin/yang and five elements are used mainly to explain the entire relationship between the human body and universe, the organization and both physiology and pathology, thus guiding clinical diagnosis and treatments.

Characteristics of Yin/Yang Theory

- mutual opposition and restriction
- mutual dependence and interaction
- wane/wax and equilibrium between yin/yang
- mutual transformation

Applications of Yin/Yang Theory in TCM

- explaining structure of the body (body type)
- explaining physiology of the body
- explaining pathology in the body
- application to clinical diagnosis and syndrome differentiation
- guiding clinical treatment and herbal application

Characteristics of Five Elements Theory

- theories based on observation of dynamic processes, functions and characteristics in the natural world
- five basic material elements: wood, fire, earth, metal and water energetic relationships within microcosm and macrocosm ("laws of five elements")
- corresponding to human body and internal organs
- movement of five elements referring to cycles: generating cycle, controlling cycle and counter-acting cycle

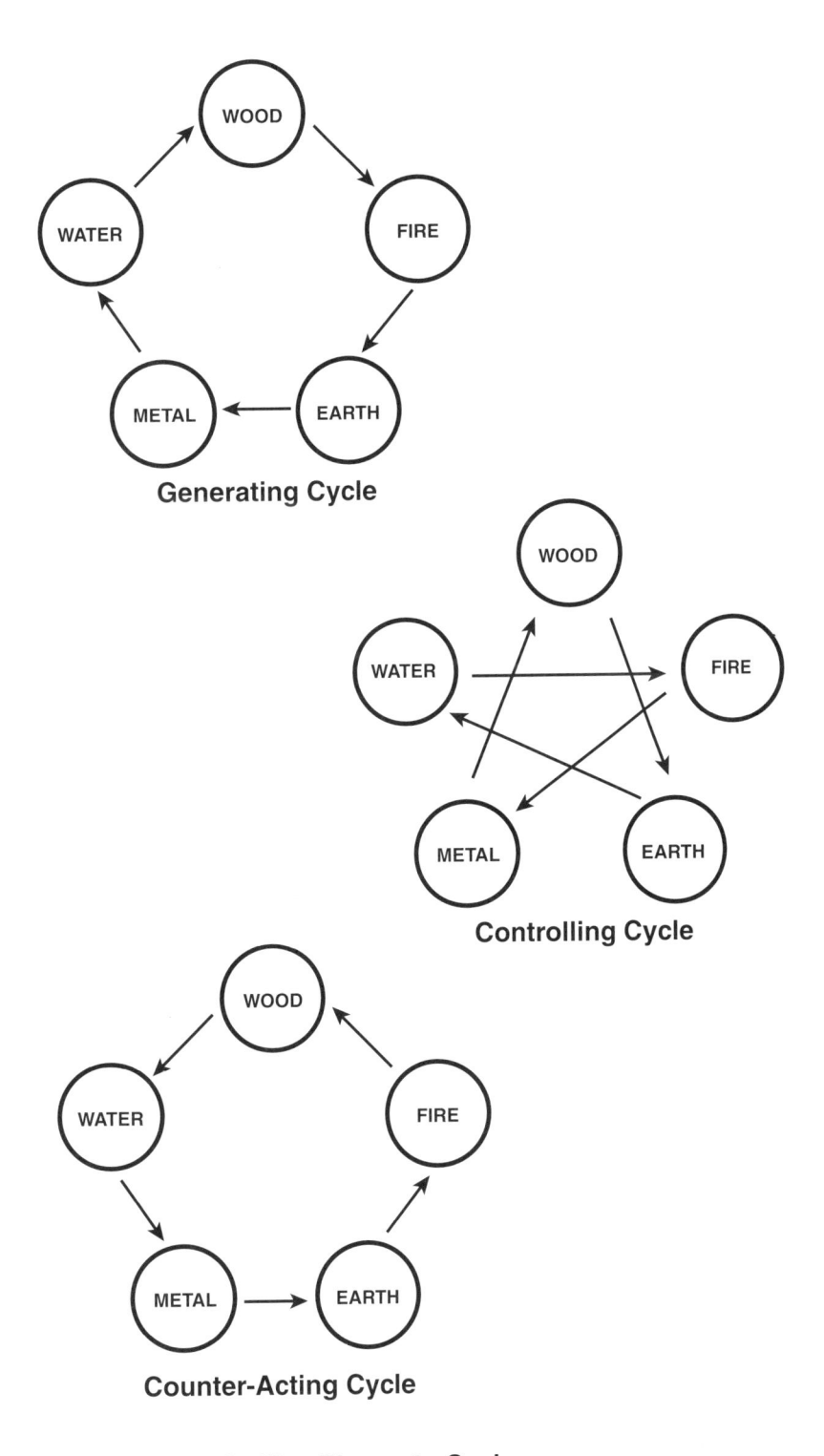

Fig. 2-1. Five Elements Cycles

Generative Cycle

- wood generates fire
- fire generates earth
- earth generates metal
- metal generates water
- water generates wood

Controlling Cycle

- wood controls earth
- earth controls water
- water controls fire
- fire controls metal
- metal controls wood

Counter-Acting Cycle

- wood counter-acts water
- water counter-acts metal
- metal counter-acts earth
- earth counter-acts fire
- fire counter-acts wood

Application of Five Elements Theory in TCM

- to differentiate the structure of the body (body type)
- to illustrate visceral functions and mutual relationships
- to identify pathogenesis and transmission
- to establish a diagnosis
- to determine principles and methods of treatment

Visceral Manifestation

Basic Concept of Visceral Manifestation

- five Zang-organs refer to deeply seated viscera in the body
- six Fu-organs refer to superficially seated viscera in the body
- studies of physiological and pathological activities of the viscera
- studies of the relationship among the viscera
- five Zang-organs: heart, lung, spleen, liver, kidney
- six Fu-organs: gall bladder, stomach, small intestine, large intestine, urinary bladder, triple heater
- extra-ordinary organs: brain, marrow, bone, vessels, uterus
- understanding of the relationships between the Zang-organs and Fu-organs is of great significance in differentiation of syndromes

Essence, Qi, Blood and Body Fluid

Essence

- pre-heaven essence: original substance of life
- post-heaven essence: extract from food
- pre-heaven and post-heaven essence: creation of vitality
- essence: root of premordial Qi (intertransformation)

Qi

- fundamental substance constituting the universe
- changes and movements of Qi producing all natural phenomena
- essential substance of the human body
- maintaining vital and functional activities of internal organs and tissues
- physiological functions of Qi: promoting, warming, defending, consolidating, transforming
- classification of Qi: primordial Qi, pectoral Qi, nutritive Qi, defensive Qi

Blood

- wet liquid circulating in vessels
- vital nutritional substance in the body
- formation of blood relies on food enzymes produced by spleen and stomach
- blood circulation nourishes and moisturizes tissues and organs
- material foundation for human mental activities

Body Fluid

- body fluid: normal secretion of viscera and tissues, saliva, gastric juice, intestinal juice, synovial fluid, tears, nasal discharge, sweat, urine
- formation, distribution and secretion of body fluid involving physiological function of viscera

Inter-Relationship among Qi, Blood and Body Fluids

- Qi and blood control vital function activities of human body
- Qi provides warmth and motive force
- blood provides nourishment and moisture
- Qi: commander of blood
- blood: mother of Qi
- importance of these relationships: for differentiation of syndromes and planning of acupuncture treatment
- deficiency of Qi: loss of body fluid
- loss of body fluid: leading to Qi deficiency
- both blood and body fluid share the function of nourishing and moisturizing
- body fluid and blood: same origin and transforming into each other

TCM Pathology

Etiology and Pathogenesis

- six climatic evils (exogenous factors): wind, cold, summer heat, dampness, dryness, fire
- pestilential evils – epidemic pathogenic invasion
- parasites
- internal injuries by seven emotions: joy, anger, melancholy, anxiety, grief, fear, terror
- improper diet and maladjustment of work and rest
- traumatic injuries
- retention of phlegm, fluid and stagnant blood

TCM Pathological Mechanism
- constitution related to congenital disposition
- disharmony of yin and yang
- struggle between Genuine Qi and Evil Qi
- factors related to age, mental state, environment, nutrition and physical activities
- disturbance of Qi and blood
- abnormal metabolism of body fluids
- dysfunction of viscera and meridians

TCM Health Prevention
- "A human body full of Genuine Qi will not be invaded by Evil Qi."
- precaution against pathogenic invasion
- endorsing eugenics for better constitution
- maintaining stability of mental activities
- promoting physical activities and leading a regular life
- providing artificial immunity (variolation to prevent small pox)
- health prevention with Chinese herbs and acupuncture

Principles of TCM Treatments
- distinguishing root vs. branch
- priority in treating root or branch
- strengthening body resistance and eliminating pathogenic factors
- regulation of yin and yang
- regulation of functions of viscera
- regulation of Qi and blood
- treatment according to seasonal conditions, local conditions and individual physical conditions

Chapter Three

Basic Meridians in Traditional Chinese Medicine

The meridians are considered to be pathways in which the Qi and blood are circulated in the human body. They are the lines connecting acupuncture points on the surface of the human body. Each meridian corresponds to a specific internal organ. In Traditional Chinese Medicine, the network of the meridians plays an important role in the diagnosis and treatment of a human body. In acupuncture, there are fourteen basic meridians, which were actually simplified from a complicated Jing-Lo system having twelve regular meridians plus the governing and conception vessels. There are three yin and three yang meridians in each limb.

In the upper limb, there are three yin meridians – lung, pericardium and heart. They originate from the trunk of the body and travel along the flexor surface of the upper extremity and end in the hand. The three yang meridians – large intestine, triple heater and small intestine – originate from the hand and travel along the extensor surface of the upper extremity and ascend to the face.

In the lower extremity, there are three yin meridians – spleen, liver and kidney. They originate from the foot, travel along the medial aspect of the lower extremity, pass along the abdomen and end in the chest. There are three yang meridians – stomach, gall bladder and urinary bladder. The stomach meridian originates from the face and travels anteriorly, passing along the chest, abdomen and the anterior aspect of the lower extremity and then ends in the foot. The gall bladder meridian originates from the face and travels laterally along the lateral aspect of the chest, abdomen and the lower extremity and ends in the foot. The urinary bladder meridian originates from the face and travels across the top of the head and then descends along the back in two lines. In the lower extremity, this meridian descends along the posterior aspect of the thigh and leg and ends in the foot.

Fourteen Classical Acupuncture Meridians

Table 3-1

	Upper Extremity	Lower Extremity	Anterior Midline of Body	Posterior Midline of Body	No. of Points
Yin	Lung (LU)				11
	Pericardium (PC)				9
	Heart (HT)				9
		Kidney (LI)			27
		Liver (LR)			14
		Spleen (SP)			21
			Conception Vessel (CV)		24
Yang	Large Intestine (LI)				20
	Triple Heater (TH)				23
	Small Intestine (SI)				19
		Stomach (ST)			45
		Gall bladder (GB)			44
		Bladder (BL)			67
				Governor Vessel (GV)	28
Total Number of Points					**361**

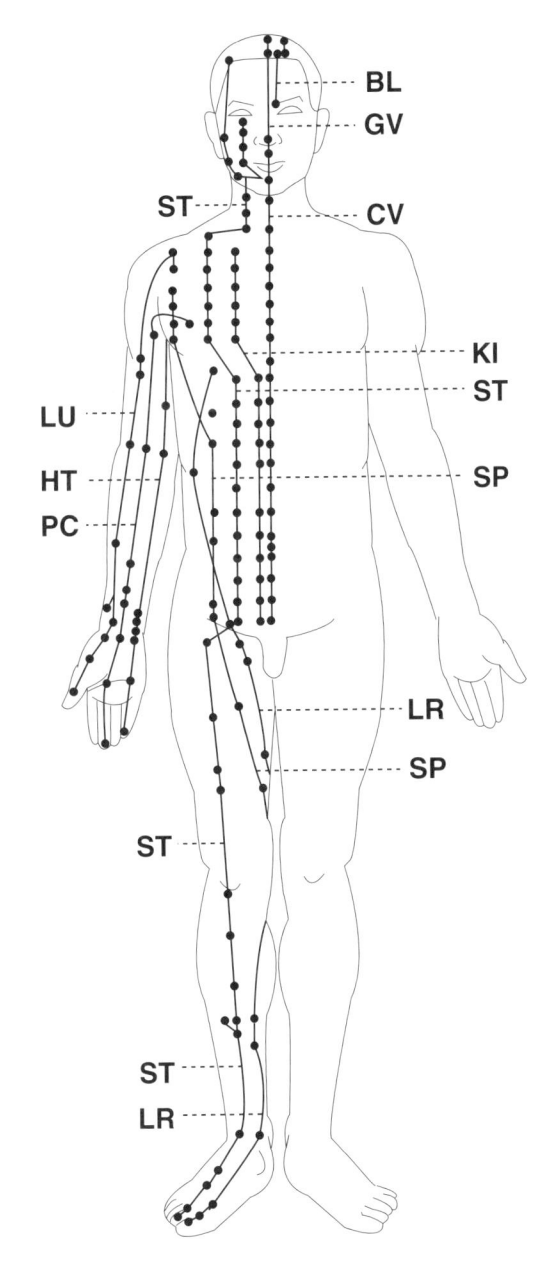

Fig. 3-1. Anterior View - Acupuncture Meridians

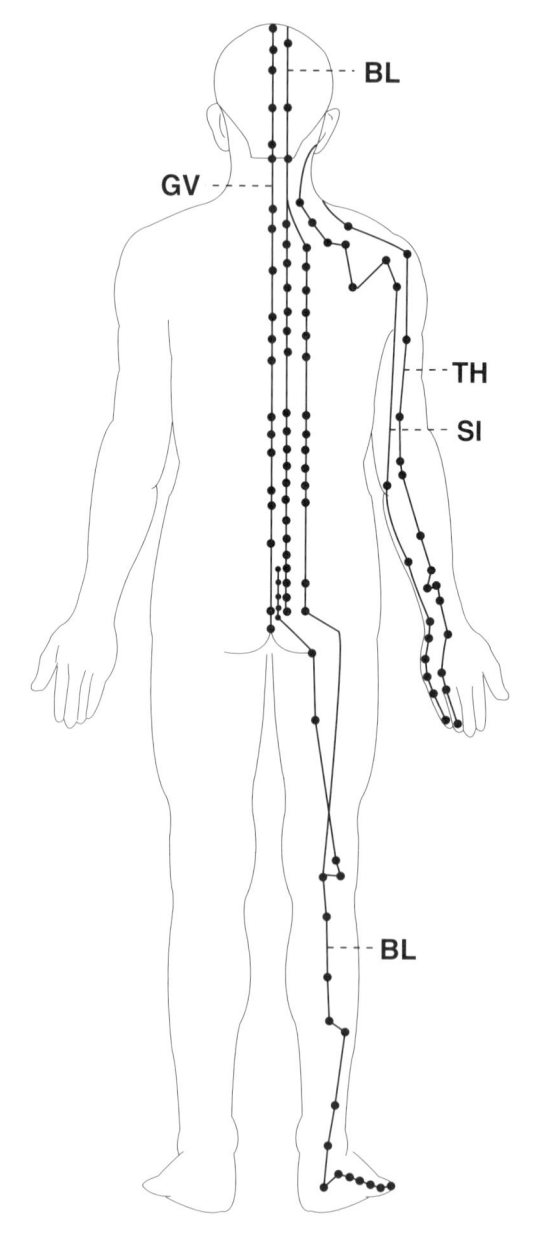

Fig. 3-2. Posterior View - Acupuncture Meridians

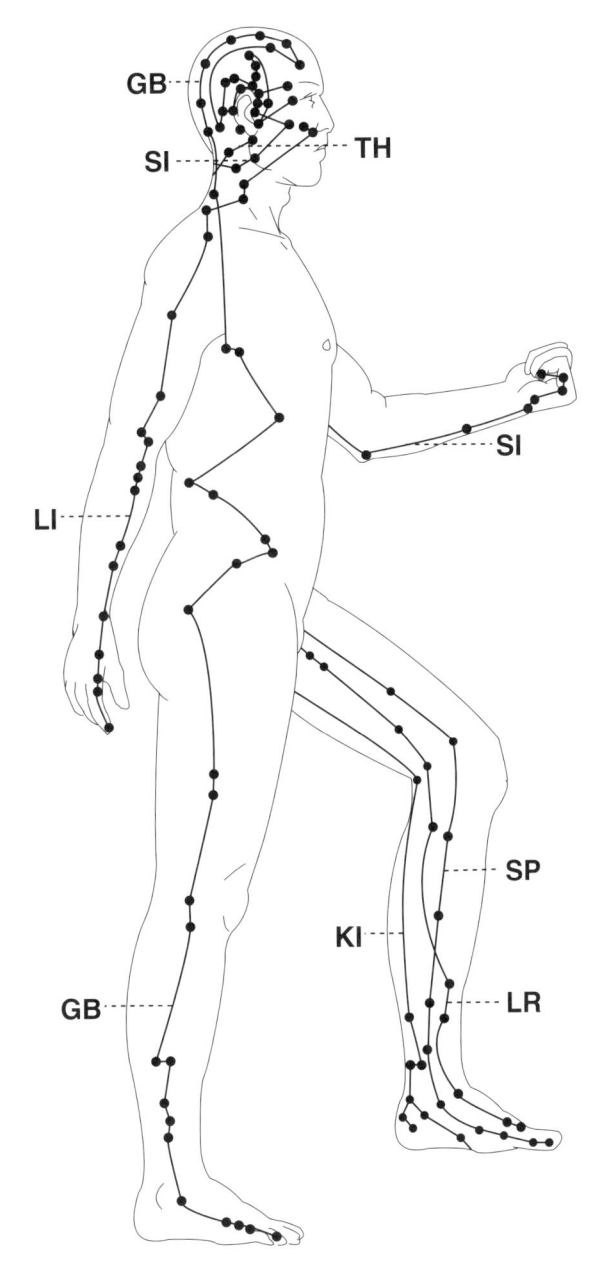

Fig. 3-3. Lateral View - Acupuncture Meridians

Chapter Four

Standard Acupuncture Nomenclature

Acupuncture has developed and evolved not only in China, but in the other countries in the world. There are many differences in nomenclature, which have given rise to various difficulties. For example, certain acupuncture points have a number of different names, while the different ways of pronouncing the Chinese characters have caused mistakes and misunderstandings.

The need for acupuncture nomenclature to be internationalized and standardized is now recognized by the acupuncturists in the world. Therefore, the resulting uniformity is expected to greatly facilitate understanding among all the acupuncturists in the world. In this way, a standard nomenclature will facilitate both the teaching and understanding of published research materials and also permit more accurate description and location of acupuncture points.

Therefore, in this book, I am following the system endorsed by the World Health Organization (WHO). The English language name of the fourteen principal meridians and their alphabetic codes are listed as follows:

Table 4-1

Principal Meridian	Alphabetic Code
Lung	LU
Large Intestine	LI
Stomach	ST
Spleen	SP
Heart	HT
Small Intestine	SI
Bladder	BL
Kidney	KI
Pericardium	PC
Triple Heater	TH
Gallbladder	GB
Liver	LR
Governor Vessel	GV
Conception Vessel	CV

List of Equivalent Alphabetic Codes of Meridian Names

Table 4-2

Meridian	Standard Code	Other Alphabetic Codes Used
Lung	LU	L, Lu, F, P
Large Intestine	LI	CO, Co, Dch, DI, Di, GI, IC, IG, Li
Stomach	ST	S, St, E, Est, M, Ma, V, W
Spleen	SP	Sp, B, BP, LP, MP, P, RP, RT, Rt
Heart	HT	H, He, HE, Ht, C, X
Small Intestine	SI	Dii, ID, IG, IT, SI, Xch
Bladder	BL	B, UB, B1, PG, V, VU
Kidney	KI	K, Ki, N, NI, Ni, R, RN, Rn, Sh
Pericardium	PC	P, CS, CX, ECs, EH, HC, Hc, KS, MC, MdH, Pe, XB
Triple Heater	TH	TE, TW, T, TB, TR, DE, SC, SJ, 3E, 3H
Gallbladder	GB	G, D, Go, VB, VF
Liver	LR	Liv, LIV, LV, Lv, LE, F, G, H
Governor Vessel	GV	DM, DU, Du, GG, Go, Gv, LG, Lg, T, TM, VG, Vg
Conception Vessel	CV	Co, Cv, J, JM, KG, Kg, REN, Ren, RM, VC, Vc

The Acupuncture Points with Alphameric Code, the Chinese Alphabet Name and the Original Han Character

Lung Meridian, LU
Shǒutàiyīn Fèijīng xué

手太陰(阴)肺經(経, 经)

LU 1	Zhōngfǔ	中府	LU 7	Lièquē	列缺
LU 2	Yúnmén	雲(云)門(门)	LU 8	Jīngqú	經(経, 经)渠
LU 3	Tiānfǔ	天府	LU 9	Tàiyuān	太淵(渊)
LU 4	Xiábái	俠(侠)白	LU 10	Yújì	魚(鱼)際(际)
LU 5	Chǐzé	尺澤(沢, 泽)	LU 11	Shàoshāng	少商
LU 6	Kǒngzuì	孔最			

Large Intestine Meridian, LI
Shǒuyángmíng Dàcháng- Jīng xué

手陽(阳)明大陽(肠)經(経, 经)

LI 1	Shāngyáng	商陽(阳)	LI 11	Qūchí	曲池
LI 2	Èrjiān	二間(间)	LI 12	Zhǒuliáo	肘髎
LI 3	Sānjiān	三間(间)	LI 13	Shǒuwǔlǐ	手五里
LI 4	Hégǔ	合谷	LI 14	Bìnào	臂臑
LI 5	Yángxī	陽(阳)谿(溪)	LI 15	Jiānyú	肩髃
LI 6	Piānlì	偏歷(歴, 历)	LI 16	Jùgǔ	巨骨
LI 7	Wēnliū	溫(温)溜	LI 17	Tiāndǐng	天鼎
LI 8	Xiàlián	下廉	LI 18	Fútū	扶突
LI 9	Shànglián	上廉	LI 19	Kǒuhéliáo	禾髎
LI 10	Shǒusānlǐ	手三里	LI 20	Yíngxiāng	迎(迎)香

Stomach Meridian, ST
Zúyángmíng Wèijīng xué

足陽(阳)明胃經(経, 经)

ST 1	Chéngqì	承泣	ST 4	Dìcāng	地倉(仓)
ST 2	Sìbái	四白	ST 5	Dàyíng	大迎
ST 3	Jùliáo	巨髎	ST 6	Jiáchē	頬(颊)車(车)

ST 7	Xiàguān	下關(関, 关)	ST 27	Dàjù	大巨
ST 8	Tóuwéi	頭(头)維(维)	ST 28	Shuǐdào	水道(道)
ST 9	Rényíng	人迎	ST 29	Guīlái	歸(帰, 归)來(来)
ST 10	Shuǐtū	水突	ST 30	Qìchōng	氣(気, 气)衝(冲)
ST 11	Qìshè	氣(気, 气)舍(舍)	ST 31	Bìguān	髀(髀)關(関, 关)
ST 12	Quēpén	缺盆	ST 32	Fútù	伏兔(兔)
ST 13	Qìhù	氣(気, 气)戶	ST 33	Yīnshì	陰(阴)市
ST 14	Kùfáng	庫(库)房	ST 34	Liángqiū	梁丘
ST 15	Wūyì	屋翳	ST 35	Dúbí	犢(犊)鼻
ST 16	Yīngchuāng	膺窓(窗)	ST 36	Zúsānlǐ	足三里
ST 17	Rǔzhōng	乳中	ST 37	Shàngjùxū	上巨虛(虚)
ST 18	Rǔgēn	乳根	ST 38	Tiáokǒu	條(条)口
ST 19	Bùróng	不容	ST 39	Xiàjùxū	下巨虛(虚)
ST 20	Chéngmǎn	承滿(満, 满)	ST 40	Fēnglóng	豐(丰)隆
ST 21	Liángmén	梁門(门)	ST 41	Jiěxī	解谿(溪)
ST 22	Guānmén	關(関, 关)門(门)	ST 42	Chōngyáng	衝(冲)陽(阳)
ST 23	Tàiyǐ	太乙	ST 43	Xiàngǔ	陷(陥)谷
ST 24	Huáròumén	滑(滑)肉門(门)	ST 44	Nèitíng	內庭
ST 25	Tiānshū	天樞(枢)	ST 45	Lìduì	厲(历)兌(兑)
ST 26	Wàilíng	外陵			

Spleen Meridian, SP
Zútàiyīn Píjīng xué

足太陰(阴)脾經(経, 经)

SP 1	Yǐnbái	隱(隐)白	SP 12	Chōngmén	衝(冲)門(门)
SP 2	Dàdū	大都	SP 13	Fǔshè	府舍(舍)
SP 3	Tàibái	太白	SP 14	Fùjié	腹結
SP 4	Gōngsūn	公孫(孙)	SP 15	Dàhéng	大橫
SP 5	Shāngqiū	商丘	SP 16	Fù'āi	腹哀
SP 6	Sānyīnjiāo	三陰(阴)交	SP 17	Shídòu	食竇(窦)
SP 7	Lòugǔ	漏谷	SP 18	Tiānxī	天谿(溪)
SP 8	Dìjī	地機(机)	SP 19	Xiōngxiāng	胸鄉(乡)
SP 9	Yīnlíngquán	陰(阴)陵泉	SP 20	Zhōuróng	周榮(栄, 荣)
SP 10	Xuèhǎi	血海(海)	SP 21	Dàbāo	大包(包)
SP 11	Jīmén	箕門(门)			

Heart Meridian, HT
Shǒushàoyīn Xīnjīng xué
手少陰(阴)心經(経,经)

HT 1	Jíquán	極(极)泉	HT 6	Yīnxì	陰(阴)郄
HT 2	Qīnglíng	青(青)靈(霊,灵)	HT 7	Shénmén	神(神)門(门)
HT 3	Shàohǎi	少海(海)	HT 8	Shàofǔ	少府
HT 4	Língdào	靈(霊,灵)道(道)	HT 9	Shàochōng	少衝(冲)
HT 5	Tōnglǐ	通(通)里			

Small Intestine Meridian, SI
Shǒutàiyáng Xiǎochángjīng xué
手太陽(阳)小腸(肠)經(経,经)

SI 1	Shàozé	少澤(沢,泽)	SI 11	Tiānzōng	天宗
SI 2	Qiángǔ	前谷	SI 12	Bǐngfēng	秉風(风)
SI 3	Hòuxī	後(后)谿(溪)	SI 13	Qūyuán	曲垣
SI 4	Wàngǔ	腕骨(骨)	SI 14	Jiānwàishū	肩外俞
SI 5	Yánggǔ	陽(阳)谷	SI 15	Jiānzhōngshū	肩中俞
SI 6	Yǎnglǎo	養(养)老	SI 16	Tiānchuāng	天窓(窗)
SI 7	Zhīzhèng	支正	SI 17	Tiānróng	天容
SI 8	Xiǎohǎi	小海(海)	SI 18	Quánliáo	顴(颧)髎
SI 9	Jiānzhēn	肩貞(贞)	SI 19	Tīnggōng	聽(聴,听)宮(宫)
SI 10	Nàoshū	臑俞			

Bladder Meridian, BL
Zútàiyáng pángguāngjīng xué
足太陽(阳)膀胱經(経,经)

BL 1	Jīngmíng	睛(睛)明	BL 8	Luòquè	絡(络)郄(却)
BL 2	Cuánzhú(Zǎnzhú)	攢(攒)竹	BL 9	Yùzhěn	玉枕
BL 3	Méichōng	眉衝(冲)	BL 10	Tiānzhù	天柱
BL 4	Qūchā(Qūchāi)	曲差	BL 11	Dàzhù	大杼
BL 5	Wǔchù	五處(処,处)	BL 12	Fēngmén	風(风)門(门)
BL 6	Chéngguāng	承光	BL 13	Fèishū	肺俞
BL 7	Tōngtiān	通(通)天	BL 14	Juéyīnshū	厥陰(阴)俞

BL 15	Xīnshū	心俞		BL 42	Pòhù	魄戶
BL 16	Dūshū	督俞		BL 43	Gāohuāng	膏肓
BL 17	Géshū	膈俞		BL 44	Shéntáng	神(神)堂
BL 18	Gānshū	肝俞		BL 45	Yìxǐ	譩(譩)譆(譆)
BL 19	Dǎnshū	膽(胆)俞		BL 46	Géguān	膈關(関,关)
BL 20	Píshū	脾俞		BL 47	Húnmén	魂門(门)
BL 21	Wèishū	胃俞		BL 48	Yánggāng	陽(阳)綱(纲)
BL 22	Sānjiāoshū	三焦俞		BL 49	Yìshè	意舍(舍)
BL 23	Shènshū	腎(肾)俞		BL 50	Wèicāng	胃倉(仓)
BL 24	Qìhǎishū	氣(気,气)海(海)俞		BL 51	Huāngmén	肓門(门)
BL 25	Dàchángshū	大腸(肠)俞		BL 52	Zhìshì	志室
BL 26	Guānyuánshū	關(関,关)元俞		BL 53	Bāohuāng	胞(胞)肓
BL 27	Xiǎochángshū	小腸(肠)俞		BL 54	Zhìbiān	秩邊(边)
BL 28	Pángguāngshū	膀胱俞		BL 55	Héyáng	合陽(阳)
BL 29	Zhōnglǔshū	中膂俞		BL 56	Chéngjīn	承筋
BL 30	Báihuánshū	白環(环)俞		BL 57	Chéngshān	承山
BL 31	Shàngliáo	上髎(髎)		BL 58	Fēiyáng	飛(飞)揚(扬)
BL 32	Cìliáo	次髎(髎)		BL 59	Fūyáng	跗陽(阳)
BL 33	Zhōngliáo	中髎(髎)		BL 60	Kūnlún	崑(昆)崙(侖,仑)
BL 34	Xiàliáo	下髎(髎)		BL 61	Púcān(Púshēn)	僕(仆)參(参)
BL 35	Huìyáng	會(会)陽(阳)		BL 62	Shēnmài	申脈(脉)
BL 36	Chéngfú	承扶		BL 63	Jīnmén	金門(门)
BL 37	Yīnmén	殷門(门)		BL 64	Jīnggǔ	京骨(骨)
BL 38	Fúxì	浮郄		BL 65	Shùgǔ	束骨(骨)
BL 39	Wěiyáng	委陽(阳)		BL 66	Zútōnggǔ	足通(通)谷
BL 40	Wěizhōng	委中		BL 67	Zhìyīn	至陰(阴)
BL 41	Fùfēn	附分				

Kidney Meridian, KI
Zúshàoyīn Shènjīng xué

足少陰(阴)腎(肾)經(経,经)

KI 1	Yǒngquán	湧(涌)泉		KI 8	Jiāoxìn	交信
KI 2	Rángǔ	然谷		KI 9	Zhùbīn	築(筑)賓(宾)
KI 3	Tàixī	太谿(溪)		KI 10	Yīngǔ	陰(阴)谷
KI 4	Dàzhōng	大鍾(钟)		KI 11	Hénggǔ	橫骨(骨)
KI 5	Shuǐquán	水泉		KI 12	Dàhè	大赫
KI 6	Zhàohǎi	照海(海)		KI 13	Qìxué	氣(気,气)穴
KI 7	Fùliū	復(复)溜		KI 14	Sìmǎn	四滿(満,满)

KI 15	Zhōngzhù	中注		KI 22	Bùláng	步廊
KI 16	Huāngshū	肓俞		KI 23	Shénfēng	神(神)封
KI 17	Shāngqū	商曲		KI 24	Língxū	靈(靈,灵)墟
KI 18	Shíguān	石關(関,关)		KI 25	Shéncáng	神(神)藏(蔵)
KI 19	Yīndū	陰(阴)都		KI 26	Yùzhōng	彧中
KI 20	Fùtōnggǔ	腹通(通)谷		KI 27	Shūfǔ	俞府
KI 21	Yōumén	幽門(门)				

Pericardium Meridian, PC
Shǒujuéyīn Xīnbāojīng xué
手厥陰(阴)心包經(経,经)

PC 1	Tiānchí	天池		PC 6	Nèiguān	内關(関,关)
PC 2	Tiānquán	天泉		PC 7	Dàlíng	大陵
PC 3	Qūzé	曲澤(沢,泽)		PC 8	Láogōng	勞(労,劳)宮(宫)
PC 4	Xīmén	郄門(门)		PC 9	Zhōngchōng	中衝(沖)
PC 5	Jiānshǐ	間(间)使				

Triple Heater Meridian, TH
Shǒushàoyáng Sānjiāojīng xué
手少陽(阳)三焦經(経,经)

TH 1	Guānchōng	關(関,关)衝(沖)		TH 13	Nàohuì	臑會(会)
TH 2	Yèmén	液門(门)		TH 14	Jiānliáo	肩髎
TH 3	Zhōngzhǔ	中渚(渚)		TH 15	Tiānliáo	天髎
TH 4	Yángchí	陽(阳)池		TH 16	Tiānyǒu	天牖
TH 5	Wàiguān	外關(関,关)		TH 17	Yìfēng	翳風(风)
TH 6	Zhīgōu	支溝(沟)		TH 18	Chìmài(Qìmài)	瘈脈(脉)
TH 7	Huìzōng	會(会)宗		TH 19	Lúxī	顱(颅)息
TH 8	Sānyángluò	三陽(阳)絡(络)		TH 20	Jiǎosūn	角孫(孙)
TH 9	Sìdú	四瀆(渎)		TH 21	Ěrmén	耳門(门)
TH 10	Tiānjǐng	天井		TH 22	Ěrhéliáo	和髎
TH 11	Qīnglěngyuān	清(清)冷(令)淵(渊)		TH 23	Sīzhúkōng	絲(丝)竹空
TH 12	Xiāoluò	消濼(泺)				

Gallbladder Meridian, GB
Zúshàoyáng Dǎnjīng xué

足少陽(阳)胆經(経, 经)

GB 1	Tóngzǐliáo	瞳子髎	GB 23	Zhéjīn	輒(辄)筋
GB 2	Tīnghuì	聽(聴, 听)會(会)	GB 24	Rìyuè	日月
GB 3	Shàngguān	上關(関, 关)	GB 25	Jīngmén	京門(门)
GB 4	Hànyàn	頷(颔)厭(厌)	GB 26	Dàimài	帶(带, 带)脈(脉)
GB 5	Xuánlú	懸(悬)顱(颅)	GB 27	Wǔshū	五樞(枢)
GB 6	Xuánlí	懸(悬)釐(厘)	GB 28	Wéidào	維(维)道(道)
GB 7	Qūbìn	曲鬢(鬓)	GB 29	Jūliáo	居髎(髎)
GB 8	Shuàigǔ	率谷	GB 30	Huántiào	環(环)跳
GB 9	Tiānchōng	天衝(冲)	GB 31	Fēngshì	風(风)市
GB 10	Fúbái	浮白	GB 32	Zhōngdú	中瀆(渎)
GB 11	Tóuqiàoyīn	頭(头)竅(窍)陰(阴)	GB 33	Xīyángguān	足(膝)陽(阳)關(関, 关)
GB 12	Wángǔ	完骨(骨)	GB 34	Yánglíngquán	陽(阳)陵泉
GB 13	Běnshén	本神(神)	GB 35	Yángjiāo	陽(阳)交
GB 14	Yángbái	陽(阳)白	GB 36	Wàiqiū	外丘(邱)
GB 15	Tóulínqì	頭(头)臨(临)泣	GB 37	Guāngmíng	光明
GB 16	Mùchuāng	目窗(窗)	GB 38	Yángfǔ	陽(阳)輔(辅)
GB 17	Zhèngyíng	正營(营, 营)	GB 39	Xuánzhōng	懸(悬)鍾(钟)
GB 18	Chénglíng	承靈(霊, 灵)	GB 40	Qiūxū	丘(坵)墟(墟)
GB 19	Nǎokōng	腦(脳, 脑)空	GB 41	Zúlínqì	足臨(临)泣
GB 20	Fēngchí	風(风)池	GB 42	Dìwǔhuì	地五會(会)
GB 21	Jiānjǐng	肩井	GB 43	Xiáxī	俠(侠)谿(溪)
GB 22	Yuānyè	淵(渊)腋	GB 44	Zúqiàoyīn	足竅(窍)陰(阴)

Liver Meridian, LR
Zújuéyīn Gānjīng xué

足厥陰(阴)肝經(経, 经)

LR 1	Dàdūn	大敦	LR 8	Qūquán	曲泉
LR 2	Xíngjiān	行間(间)	LR 9	Yīnbāo	陰(阴)包(包)
LR 3	Tàichōng	太衝(冲)	LR 10	Zúwǔlǐ	足五里
LR 4	Zhōngfēng	中封	LR 11	Yīnlián	陰(阴)廉
LR 5	Lígōu	蠡溝(沟)	LR 12	Jímài	急脈(脉)
LR 6	Zhōngdū	中都	LR 13	Zhāngmén	章門(门)
LR 7	Xīguān	膝關(关, 关)	LR 14	Qīmén	期門(门)

Governor Vessel Meridian, GV
Dūmài xué

督脈(脉)經(経,经)

GV 1	Chángqiáng	長(长)強	GV 15	Yǎmén	瘂(哑)門(门)
GV 2	Yāoshū	腰俞	GV 16	Fēngfǔ	風(风)府
GV 3	Yāoyángguān	腰陽(阳)關(関,关)	GV 17	Nǎohù	腦(脑,脑)戶
GV 4	Mìngmén	命門(门)	GV 18	Qiángjiān	強間(间)
GV 5	Xuánshū	懸(悬)樞(枢)	GV 19	Hòudǐng	後(后)頂(顶)
GV 6	Jǐzhōng	脊中	GV 20	Bǎihuì	百會(会)
GV 7	Zhōngshū	中樞(枢)	GV 21	Qiándǐng	前頂(顶)
GV 8	Jīnsuō	筋縮(缩)	GV 22	Xìnhuì	顖(囟)會(会)
GV 9	Zhìyáng	至陽(阳)	GV 23	Shàngxīng	上星
GV 10	Língtái	靈(靈,灵)臺(台)	GV 24	Shéntíng	神(神)庭
GV 11	Shéndào	神(神)道(道)	GV 25	Sùliáo	素髎
GV 12	Shēnzhù	身柱	GV 26	Shuǐgōu	水溝(沟)
GV 13	Táodào	陶道(道)	GV 27	Duìduān	兌端
GV 14	Dàzhuī	大椎	GV 28	Yínjiāo	齦(龈)交

Conception Vessel Meridian, CV
Rénmài xué

任脈(脉)經(経,经)

CV 1	Huìyīn	會(会)陰(阴)	CV 14	Jùquè	巨闕(阙)
CV 2	Qūgǔ	曲骨(骨)	CV 15	Jiūwěi	鳩(鸠)尾
CV 3	Zhōngjí	中極	CV 16	Zhōngtíng	中庭
CV 4	Guānyuán	關(関,关)元	CV 17	Tánzhōng	膻中
CV 5	Shímén	石門(门)		(Shāozhōng)	
CV 6	Qìhǎi	氣(気,气)海(海)	CV 18	Yùtáng	玉堂
CV 7	Yīnjiāo	陰(阴)交	CV 19	Zǐgōng	紫宮(宫)
CV 8	Shénquè	神(神)闕(阙)	CV 20	Huágài	華(华)蓋(盖)
CV 9	Shuǐfēn	水分	CV 21	Xuánjī	璇璣(玑)
CV 10	Xiàwǎn	下脘	CV 22	Tiāntū	天突
CV 11	Jiànlǐ	建里	CV 23	Liánquán	廉泉
CV 12	Zhōngwǎn	中脘	CV 24	Chéngjiāng	承漿(浆)
CV 13	Shàngwǎn	上脘			

Chapter Five

Acupuncture as a Physical Therapy

Having studied acupuncture for the past forty years, I believe that the main functions and benefits of acupuncture can be summarized as follows:

- normalization of autonomic nervous dysfunction
- control of pain
- anti-inflammation
- surgical analgesia
- control of addictions
- regeneration

Throughout its history, acupuncture has been used most extensively to normalize autonomic nervous dysfunction and control pain. Its use as a surgical analgesia and for the control of drug addiction only started in the late 1950's. In the past few years, research has been carried out on acupuncture and tissue regeneration. When acupuncture was introduced to North America, its effectiveness in the control of pain was the most attractive element for Western medical scientists (particularly after endorphin was discovered in the 1960's). Since then, scientific research has been done on acupuncture and its effect on endorphins and other neurotransmitters. Within the past thirty years, there have been hundreds of scientific papers published on this aspect of acupuncture alone. Why are Western medical scientists so interested in the pain control function of acupuncture? The answer is simple: despite Western medical science's rapid advances in many areas, doctors and patients are, in many cases, still looking for an effective treatment of pain without the deleterious side-effects of many Western conventional methods of pain control.

Let us review the major areas of pain management available through Western conventional medicine:

- surgical management
- anesthetic management
- chemical management – medications
- physical management
- psychological management

Surgical management of pain involves mostly surgery of the nervous system. Its outcome can be good but often results in the sacrifice of some normal human bodily function. Therefore, this form of management tends to be used as a last resort.

The effect of the anesthetic management is often temporary in a large number of cases.

Psychological management is effective in select patients.

In physical management, there are many physical stimuli that can alleviate pain. Some modalities are more effective than the others and there are obvious differences in the extent of the results. If we consider that heat, cold and some other primary remedies are physical therapeutic modalities, the history of physical management goes back many thousands of years. However, formal physical therapy was not started until the eighteenth century. More organized electrotherapy, such as galvanism, faradism, short wave diathermy and microwave therapy started to gain popularity after World War II.

Norman Shealy, an American neurosurgeon, pioneered dorsal column stimulation. As a by-product, he also helped to develop the TENS stimulator (transcutaneous electrical nerve stimulation). As a point of interest, at this time, electro-acupuncture was also being used. In fact, the components of the electro-acupuncture stimulator are almost identical to the TENS stimulator.

The Definition of Acupuncture

Acupuncture needle + the human body = therapeutic effect.

An acupuncture needle is a physical stimulus and, by virtue of this fact, acupuncture is a **physical therapy**. Electro-acupuncture is an **electrotherapy**.

I would like to make a general distinction between most of the physical therapeutic modalities and acupuncture as a physical therapy. Acupuncture is different from other physical therapeutic modalities because it is an **invasive technique** bypassing the skin barrier. Perhaps, in part because of this feature, acupuncture is not only more effective in alleviation of pain but also offers other desirable effects.

A Comparison of Electrotherapy Methods

Table 5-1

Frequency	Intensity	Skin	Barrier
Galvanism	20 cycles/second	High	Yes
Faradism	50-100 cycles/second	High	Yes
Short-wave Diathermy	27.12 megacycles/second	High	Yes
Ultrasound	0.8-1 megacycles/ second	High	Yes
Microwave	2456 megacycles/second	High	Yes
Interferential	4100-4000 = 100 cycles/second	Low	Yes
Transcutaneous Electrical Nerve Stimulation (TENS)	0-300 cycles/second	Low	Yes
Electro-acupuncture (PENS)	0-300 cycles/second	Low	No

A few years before the discovery of endorphins, some early researchers of acupuncture speculated on the mechanisms by which acupuncture works. They noted that the acupuncture needle is inserted into the human body and should thus be considered a foreign body. Accordingly, they conjectured, the human body ought to have a reaction to this foreign body. This speculation has now been confirmed in studies that have identified leukocytosis and an increase of eosinophils in the human blood after acupuncture treatments. This phenomenon can best be explained as an **immunological response**. Researchers also speculated that since the acupuncture needle creates a micro-injury that the body might, in spite of the minute damage to its tissue, have a regenerative response. Other physical modalities would not evoke this same type of **regenerative response** because they use, with respect to the skin, non-invasive techniques.

One other thing that could make acupuncture preferable to other physical modalities for particular problems is that it has an anti-inflammatory function. With respect to inflammation, the following clinical benefits are commonly observed:

- subsidence of redness
- subsidence of elevated local temperature
- subsidence of pain and swelling
- increase of physical function

Clearly these clinical observations lead one to conclude that acupuncture not only functions to reduce pain but also to reduce inflammation. Acupuncture is then not only an **analgesic** but also an **anti-inflammatory** treatment.

Chapter Six

Biochemical Mechanism of Acupuncture

In dealing with musculo-skeletal disorders, we should ideally achieve the following goals:

- analgesia
- anti-inflammation and restoration of physical functions
- normalization of autonomic nervous dysfunctions
- regeneration

Acupuncture is the most ideal therapeutic modality to help in achieving these goals.

Acupuncture Analgesia

Acupuncture involves a physical stimulus. The physical stimulus produced by the acupuncture needle as it is inserted into the human body generates an impulse that travels (either with or without the means of an electrical current) to the nervous system of the human body. Peripheral nerves are depolarized and there are responses from different levels of the nervous centers. The pathway of the impulse produced by the acupuncture stimulus, most likely, proceeds through the following:

- peripheral nerves
- spinal nerves
- spinal cord
- mid-brain
- hypothalamus
- thalamus
- cerebral cortex

In all these nervous structures, biochemical interactions occur that involve different neurotransmitters and hormones.

There have been a large number of modern scientific studies on the nature of acupuncture analgesia. According to Professor Bruce Pomeranz, a world-renowned acupuncture researcher at the University of Toronto, Canada, acupuncture needles stimulate type two and type three muscle afferent nerves or A-delta fibres, sending impulses to the anterolateral track of the spinal cord. The impulses advance further to either one or all of three centers – the spinal cord, the mid-brain and the pituitary hypothalamic complex.

Overall, the biochemical interactions can be summarized as the follows:

Spinal Cord Level

- interaction with substantia gelatinosa cell
- endorphinergic cell releases enkephalin or endorphin
- GABA potentiates acupuncture effects

Mid-Brain Level

- PAG cells are excited to release enkephalin
- Raphe nucleus cells release serotonin and norepinephrine

Hypothalamus Pituitary Complex

- Beta-endorphin is released into CSF and blood
- ACTH is concomitantly released, increasing cortisol level

Brain Level

- acupuncture increases serotonin in the brain – both synthesis and utilization are accelerated; central acetylcholine takes part in mediating acupuncture analgesia
- acupuncture causes significant lowering of the cerebro-norepinephrine content by stimulating its increased utilization
- acupuncture increases CSF and blood level of opiate-like substances

- GABA is antagonistic to acupuncture effect in brain
- central neurotransmitters help to exert descending control in the spinal cord

Anti-Inflammation and Restoration of Physical Function

Acupuncture Anti-Inflammation

The cardinal features of inflammation are:

- erythemia
- swelling
- elevation of local temperature
- pain
- physical dysfunction

Acupuncture treatment generates the following changes in the cardinal features of inflammation:

- disappearance of erythemia
- subsidence of swelling
- normalization of local temperature
- relief of pain
- restoration of physical function

The human body has its own anti-inflammatory functions and it seems clear that acupuncture facilitates these. The physiological mechanism may be explained as follows:

1. Peripheral Anti-Inflammatory Mechanism of Acupuncture

Inflammation is a host defense against pathogenic invasion. Mast cells exist in all vascularized tissues, predominately around arterioles. Mast cells release inflammatory mediators involving different peptides, including IGE, substance p, VIP, CGRP and CCK, etc. Inflammation is produced by interactions between white blood cells and plasma components. In 1992, Kada reported that inflammation can be modulated by sensory nerve stimulation, which is, in effect, a form of acupuncture.

2. Central Anti-Inflammatory Mechanism of Acupuncture

The central anti-inflammatory function of acupuncture may depend on the production of ACTH in the pituitary gland. During acupuncture stimulation, nerve impulses reach the hypothalamus, where releasing factor is sent to the pituitary gland, facilitating the release of ACTH from the anterior pituitary gland. In turn, ACTH increases cortisol production in the adrenal gland. Cortisol is an endogenous, powerful anti-inflammatory biochemical.

Normalization of Autonomic Nervous Dysfunction

The autonomic nervous system is a subdivision of the efferent portion of the peripheral nervous system. With acupuncture stimulus, impulses also reach (depending on the location of the acupuncture point) either the sympathetic division or the parasympathetic division of the nervous system. Autonomic nervous functions involve the biochemical interactions of two neurotransmitters – norepinephrine or acetylcholine. The function of the autonomic nervous system is to regulate effectors in order to maintain or restore the homeostasis of the human body. Autonomic nervous functions are influenced by impulses from the autonomic centers. The control centers are as follows:

- cerebral cortex
- hypothalamus
- mid-brain
- spinal cord
- extremities

Both sympathetic and parasympathetic divisions are tonically active, conducting impulses continuously to autonomic effectors. The interaction and balance of the neurotransmitters maintain the homeostasis.

Acupuncture stimulus brings about changes in the content or turn-over rate of the neurotransmitters – norepinephrine and acetylcholine. As a result, acupuncture normalizes autonomic nervous dysfunctions.

Acupuncture Regeneration

It has been commonly observed that acupuncture promotes regeneration and healing. Electromyographical studies have shown that acupuncture can enhance recovery from traumatic peripheral nerve injury even when the nerve and the muscles are partially denervated.

In the 1970's, Dr. Robert Becker started to use electrical stimulus for the regeneration of bone. Evidence suggests that physical stimulus can mend bones and possibly help to regenerate human limbs or even brain tissue. Studies have shown that there is an electrical field along acupuncture meridian pathways and that electrical stimulation promotes tissue regeneration and the healing of bone fractures. Historically, it has been evident that the human body requires "touch" in order to produce growth. The idea that touch can heal is an ancient belief – acupuncture provides a sort of "inner touch".

References

1. Becker RO, Selden G: The Body Electric. New York, Quill, 1985, pp 233-8.

2. Becker RO, Selden G: The Stimulating Current, Part 2. In Becker RO, Selden G (eds): The Body Electric. New York, Quill, 1985, pp 77-160.

3. Brattberg G: Acupuncture therapy for tennis elbow. Pain 16:285-288, 1983.

4. Bullock ML, Culliton PD, Olander RT: Controlled trial of acupuncture for severe recidivist alcoholism. Lancet 1:1435-1439, 1989.

5. Carley PJ, Wainapel SF: Electrotherapy for acceleration of wound healing: Low intensity direct current. Arch Phys Med Rehabil 66:443-446, 1985

6. Chang HT: Integrative action of thalamus in the process of acupuncture for analgesia. Scientia Sinia 16, 1973.

7. Cheng RS, McKibbin LS: Electroacupuncture elevates blood cortisol levels in naïve horses, sham treatment has no effect. Int J Neurosci 10:95-97, 1980.

8. Cheng R, Pomeranz B: Electroacupuncture analgesia is mediated by stereospecific opiate receptors and is reversed by antagonists of type I receptors. Life Sci 26:631-638, 1980.

9. Christensen BV, Iuhl IU, Vilbek H, et al: Acupuncture treatment of severe knee osteoarthritis: A long-term study. Acta Anaesthesiol Scand 36:519-525, 1992.

10. Cho ZH, Chung SC, Jones JP, et al: New findings of the correlation between acupoints and corresponding brain cortices using functional MRI. Proc Natl Acad Sci USA 95:2670-2673, 1998.

11. Coan R, Wong G, Coan PL: The acupuncture treatment of neck pain: A randomized controlled study. Am J Chin Med 9:326-332, 1982.

12. Gunn CC: Neuropathic pain-A new theory for chronic pain of intrinsic origin. Annals of the Royal College of Physicians & Surgeons of Canada, 1989.

13. Gunn CC: Treating Myofascial Pain: Intramuscular Stimulation (IMS) for Myofascial Pain Syndromes of Neuropathic Origin. Multidisciplinary Pain Center, University of Washington Medical School, 1990, p 7.

14. Gunn CC, Milbrandt WE, Little AS, et al: Dry needling of muscle motor points for chronic low-back pain: A randomized clinical trial with long-term follow-up. Spine 5:279-291, 1980.

15. Han JS, et al: The role of central 5-hydroxytryptamine in acupuncture analgesia. Scientia Sinia 22:91-104, 1979.

16. Hao J, Zhao C, Cao S, et al: Electric acupuncture treatment of peripheral nerve injury. J Tradit Chin Med 15:114-117, 1995.

17. Hinsenkamp M., Burny F: Electromagnetic stimulation of bone growth and repair. Acta Orthop Scand 196:53, 1982.

18. Kho H-G, Robertson EN: The mechanisms of acupuncture analgesia: Review and update. American Journal of Acupuncture 25:261-281, 1997.

19. Lundeberg T: Peripheral effects of sensory nerve stimulation (acupuncture) in inflammation and ischemia. Scand I Rehabil Med Suppl 29:61-86, 1993.

20. Oleson TD, Kroening RJ, Bresler DE: An experimental evaluation of auricular diagnosis: The somatotopic mapping of musculoskeletal pain at ear acupuncture points. Pain 8:217-229, 1980.

21. Pomeranz B: Electroacupuncture and transcutaneous electrical nerve stimulation. In Stux G, Pomeranz B (eds): Basics of Acupuncture, ed 2. Berlin, Springer-Verlag, 1991, pp 250-260.

22. Pomeranz B: Scientific basis of acupuncture. In Stux G, Pomeranz B (eds): Acupuncture Textbook and Atlas, Berlin, Springer-Verlag, 1987, pp 1-34.

23. Spadaro JA: Electrically stimulated bone growth in animals and man. Clin Orthop 122:325-332, 1977.

24. Tasker RR: Deafferentation. In Wall PD, Melzack R: Textbook of Pain. Churchill Livingstone, Longman Group, 1984, p 119.

25. Travell JG, Simons DG: Brachialis Muscle. In Travell JG, Simons DG (eds): Myofascial Pain and Dysfunction The Trigger Point Manual, vol 1. Baltimore, Williams and Wilkins, 1983, p 456.

26. Travell JG, Simons DG: Myofascial Pain and Dysfunction The Trigger Point Manual. Baltimore, Williams and Wilkins, vol 1, 1983; vol 2, 1992.

27. Vincent C, Lewith G: Placebo controls for acupuncture studies. J R Soc Med 88:199-202, 1995.

Chapter Seven

Acupuncture in Pain Management

Pain is one of the most debilitating experiences known to man, yet it can be simply divided into two stages or types – acute and chronic. In the acute stage, pain serves as an alarm system, warning us that something biologically harmful is happening to our body. In the chronic stage, pain often causes both intense physical and emotional stress. This division is simple yet pain can sometimes be very puzzling. So, for instance, its signals may not manifest themselves even when serious and extensive injuries have occurred. And yet, at other times, pain signals manifest themselves, but no significant injury is found that can account for either their presence or intensity.

It has been reported that chronic pain alone costs the American people more than one hundred billion dollars per year. Both the economic burden and physiological dysfunction produced by pain have created serious national and international health problems. Accordingly, the mechanism of pain has been investigated by professional disciplines covering the fields of psychology, biology and medicine. The contributions made by these disciplines towards understanding the mechanisms of pain have often given rise to conflicting observations and an overabundance of interpretations.

1. Acute Pain

In most circumstances, acute pain starts immediately after trauma. Nevertheless, there are occasions when the pain signals are deferred for hours after an injury. I have seen a large number of motor vehicle accident patients during my years of clinical experience. A number of these patients reported that they did not experience any pain or physical dysfunction immediately after the motor vehicle accident. Furthermore, some of these patients had been examined by an emergency room physician who found no evidence of any injury at the time immediately following the patients' accidents. Nevertheless, some six to twelve hours later, these patients started to experience pain in the neck, which became so severe that they were eventually immobilized or disabled. At this time, they were diagnosed with severe whiplash. This type of phenomenon is somewhat confusing.

My explanation is that it is related to the biochemical interactions of the human body. The body produces biochemicals in order to manage emergent pain. Most likely, it recognizes the motor vehicle accident as a crisis. During the crisis, the body will send impulses to the hypothalamus, which then produces releasing factor. As a result, ACTH and beta-endorphins are secreted concomitantly by the anterior pituitary gland. These substances with-hold the pain and inflammation temporarily.

In the acute pain stage, it is a common medical practice to use methylprednisolone to reduce pain and swelling resulting from head injuries. This is one place, among many, that acupuncture treatment can be used as an ideal alternative because the acupuncture stimulus can produce impulses that will reach the hypothalamus, which will, in turn, trigger processes whereby pain and swelling will be reduced. With intensive and continuous acupuncture treatments, inflammation will quickly subside and an earlier recovery will result.

2. Chronic Pain

In general, a diagnosis of chronic pain is made once a person has suffered from pain for a period of more than six to eight weeks. Sometimes definitions of chronic pain are based on underlying pathology. For instance, pain is considered chronic when it is still present yet the pathology which initially produced the pain has healed. At other times, chronic pain is diagnosed when there is a permanent pathological condition present, such as malignancy. At any rate, persistent pain is a distinct medical entity different from acute pain in a number of aspects. For example, other factors, such as psychological, social and economical factors, often become more important in the management of chronic pain than they are in short term care of acute pain.

Pain sufferers are often prescribed pain medications, including analgesics and narcotics. These medications can produce a number of problems. Endogenous biochemical pain control relies on a **physiological negative feedback** mechanism. Unfortunately, taking exogenous narcotics can reduce or even shut down the production of endogenous pain-relief biochemicals. This interference in the natural physiological negative feedback loop can also affect other related hypothalamic functions. As a result, the patient might not only suffer from chronic pain but also chronic pain affective disorders, such as depression, sleep disturbance, constipation, fatigue and loss of libido. These disorders become a part of a chronic pain syndrome. Patients experiencing this syndrome may develop a tolerance for the narcotics that they are using and, as a result, increase their narcotic intake, which in turn produces further side-effects, making the chronic pain syndrome worse and producing a vicious cycle of dependency and disorder. Chronic pain syndrome is debilitating and its victims are often beset with an ever increasing sense of helplessness, hopelessness and meaninglessness. Chronic pain can become intolerable and it almost always presents a special challenge to the health professionals and their patients.

In dealing with chronic pain or chronic pain syndrome, acupuncture is an excellent and, in many cases, preferable therapeutic modality. It controls pain so that the patients can reduce and eventually discontinue their narcotic medications. Acupuncture is known to be an effective tool in order to deal with narcotic addiction and its withdrawal symptoms. Acupuncture can also be used to help control depression and other problems, such as fatigue, constipation, loss of libido and sleep disorders (which, as noted, are potential side-effects of a dependence on narcotics).

Good pain management requires a holistic approach. Some pain can be eliminated and the patient can be cured. Unfortunately, some pain cannot be removed and some patients' problems are incurable. Yet, in dealing with pain, we should keep two fundamental goals in mind:

- to control and/or eliminate the patient's pain
- to help the patient's body cope with pain

Acupuncture Pain Management

Table 7-1

	Goals
Elimination of pain pathology	1. Control pain. 2. Reduce inflammation. 3. Restore somatic and autonomic functions. 4. Help to regenerate.
Coping with pain	1. Facilitate patient's own pain-relief mechanism by spinal or brain stimulation. (see Fig. 7-1) 2. Control narcotic side-effects (acupuncture detoxification). 3. Deal with chronic pain affective disorders (depression, insomnia, fatigue, etc.). 4. Break pain viscous cycles and promote patient's general health.

The Brain Stimulation for Pain

Table 7-2

Site of Stimulation	Acupuncture Point	Location
Medulla Oblongata	GV 26	superior to midpoint of philtrum
Hypothalamus and Mid-brain	GV 24.5	midpoint between medial ends of eyebrows
Cortex (Frontal Lobe)	GV 24	midline of head, 0.5 cun posterior to anterior hair margin
Thalamus	Thalamus point	midpoint between GV 24.5 and GV 24
Cortex, Thalamus, Hypothalamus	GV 20	on midline of head, 7 cun anterior to posterior hair margin, midpoint on a line connecting apex of two auricles
Mid-brain	GV 19	on midline of head, 5.5 cun anterior to posterior hair margin
Cerebellum, Pons	GV 18	on midline of head, 4 cun anterior to posterior hair margin
Cerebellum, Pons	GV 17	on midline of head, immediately anterior to occipital tuberance
Medulla Oblongata	GV 16	midline of spine, between C 1 posterior tubercle and occipital bone

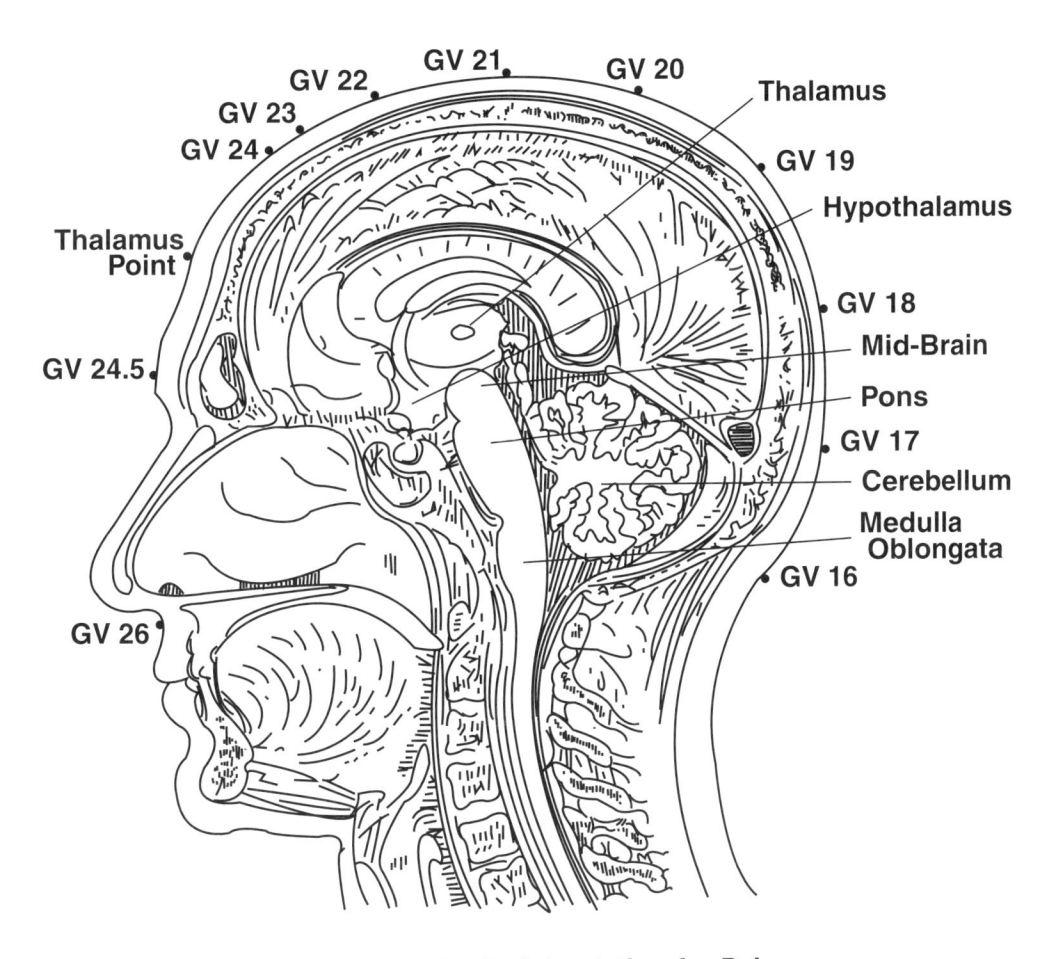

Fig. 7-1. The Brain Stimulation for Pain

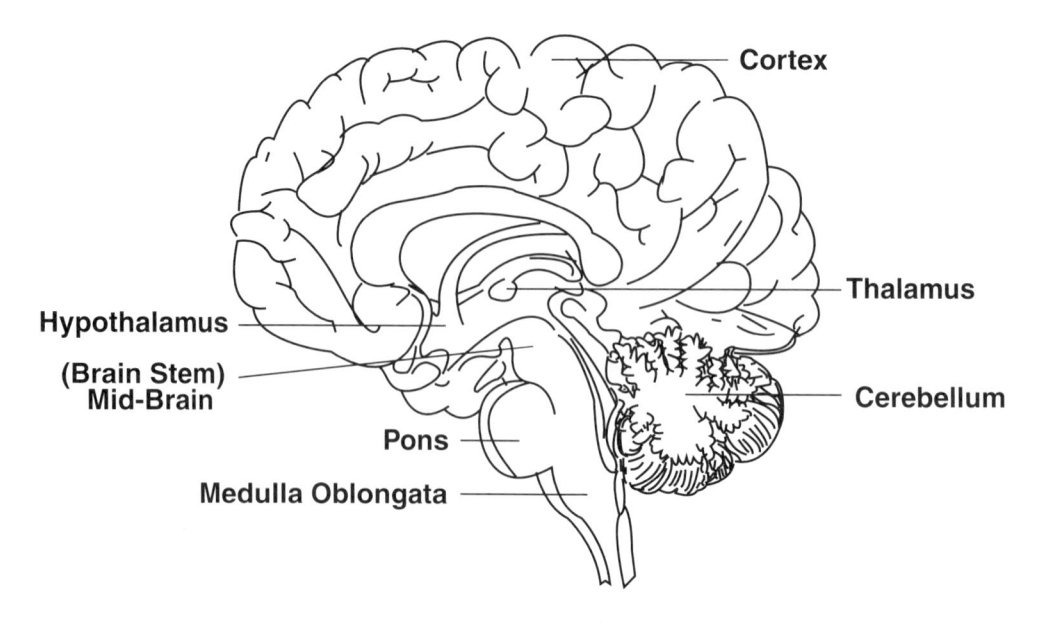

Fig. 7-2. Sagittal Section of Brain

Pathological Pain and Physiological Pain

Acupuncture can be used to treat pathological pain, particularly that involving inflammation. Acupuncture can also be used to control physiological pain, and hence its use as a surgical analgesic. In China, some surgical operations are performed with acupuncture alone, without conventional Western anesthesia. Acupuncture has been shown to abolish pain sensation while preserving the patient's sensations of touch, temperature and vibration.

Since acupuncture has been found to be effective in helping both pathological and physiological pain, a complete and sophisticated therapeutic plan, including acupuncture therapy, will better meet the needs of patients with severe, chronic pain.

Chapter Eight

The Acupuncture Treatment

The definition of acupuncture is:

acupuncture needle + human body = therapeutic effect.

Therefore, the acupuncture treatment consists of two components: the acupuncture needle and the human body.

Acupuncture has a history of more than three thousand years. Of course, there was no metal in the beginning. The Chinese people, therefore, used different kinds of sharp objects, such as sharpened animal bones or bamboo sticks. Gold and silver needles were used after the discovery of metals. It was believed that gold needles were excitative and silver, sedative. However, within the past fifty years, only stainless steel needles have been used.

I still remember that forty years ago, I used to boil the acupuncture needles for reuse. Later, I purchased an ultrasound sterilizer and a small autoclave for cleaning and sterilizing the needles. When I was practicing in the hospitals, I was able to send them to the Central Supply Department of the hospital and they were then returned as a sterilized tray. Actually, this procedure is very practical and convenient if one has access to any hospital. About fifteen years ago, the disposable acupuncture needles came onto the market. Since then, I have been using only disposable needles.

Today, the disposable needles are made of stainless steel with either a plastic or steel handle. The needles are sterilized, individually packed and come with a plastic guiding tube.

The disposable needles come in different diameters and lengths: the diameters generally range from 0.12 mm to 0.25 mm. and the lengths between 10 mm. to 80 mm. Acupuncture needles are of different lengths because the depth of the needle insertion is varied from point to point. For some of the acupuncture points, the depth can be as shallow as one-eighth of an inch and for some others, the depth can be more than three inches. In my experience, I have found that a needle of larger diameter does not necessarily produce a greater therapeutic effect. I personally prefer fine needles: the finer the needle, the more comfortable the patient feels. A "no pain, no gain" approach definitely does not apply to this kind of treatment. I prefer a deep insertion of the needle into the upper and lower extremities: a deep insertion allows a closer contact to stimulable neuro-anatomical structures.

Acupuncture Body Landmarks and Finger Measurement

There are two kinds of **body landmarks** used in acupuncture – non-mobile and mobile. The non-mobile landmarks always remain the same, such as bones, hairline, eyebrows, facial organs, nipples, axilla, nails, umbilicus, etc. The mobile landmarks can be changeable, such as skin creases, muscles, tendons, joints, etc.

Body units (proportional measurements) are measured in different parts of the body. Each unit is based on either the patient's finger measurement or equal divisions of an individual body part of the patient. The unit of measurement is called *cun* in Chinese.

Body Units (Proportional Measurements)

Table 8-1

Head and Neck	midpoint of glabella (GV 24.5) to anterior hair margin	3	cun
	anterior hair margin to posterior hair margin	12	cun
	posterior hair margin to midpoint between C 7 and T 1 spinous processes (GV 14)	3	cun
	between corners of anterior hair margins (ST 8)	9	cun
	between mastoid processes (GB 12)	9	cun
Thorax & Abdomen	between the nipples	8	cun
	suprasternal notch (CV 22) to xyphoid process	9	cun
	Xyphoid process to midpoint of umbilicus (CV 8)	8	cun

Thorax & Abdomen	midpoint of umbilicus (CV 8) to upper margin of symphysis pubis (CV 2)	5 cun
	axillary crease to tip of 11th rib	12 cun
	anterior superior iliac spine to upper margin of symphysis pubis (CV 2)	6 cun
Back	medial border of scapula to midline of spine	3 cun
	sacroiliac joint (Dimple of Venus) to midline of spine	2 cun
Upper Extremity	transverse axillary fold to cubital crease	9 cun
	cubital crease to transverse wrist crease	12 cun
Lower Extremity	upper margin of greater trochanter to middle of patella	19 cun
	middle of patella to tip of lateral malleolus	16 cun
	upper margin of symphysis pubis to upper border of medial epicondyle of femur	18 cun
	medial condyle of tibia to tip of medial malleolus	13 cun

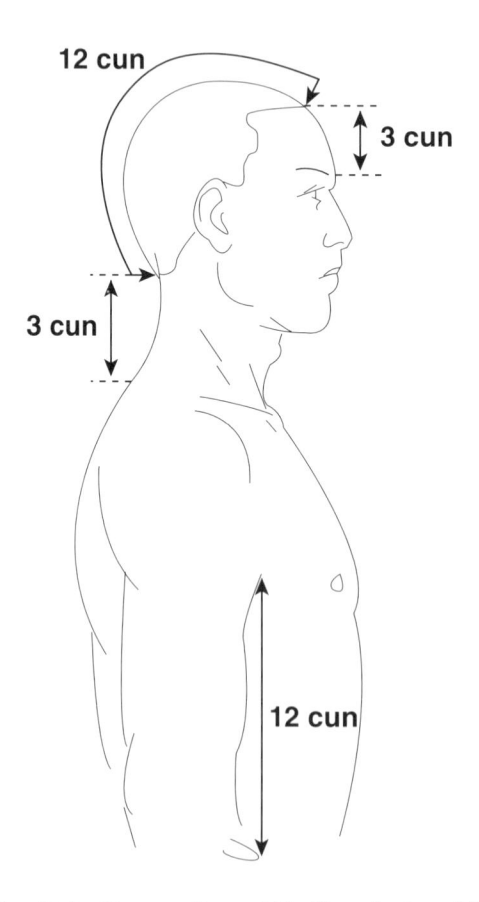

Fig. 8-1. Proportional Units - Lateral View

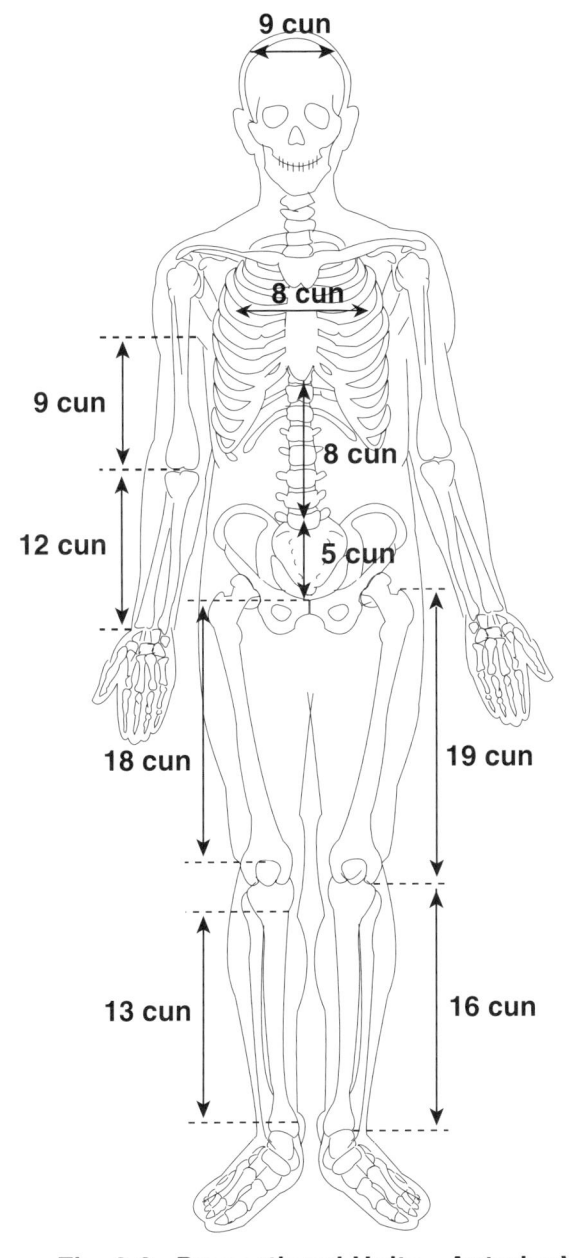

Fig. 8-2. Proportional Units - Anterior View

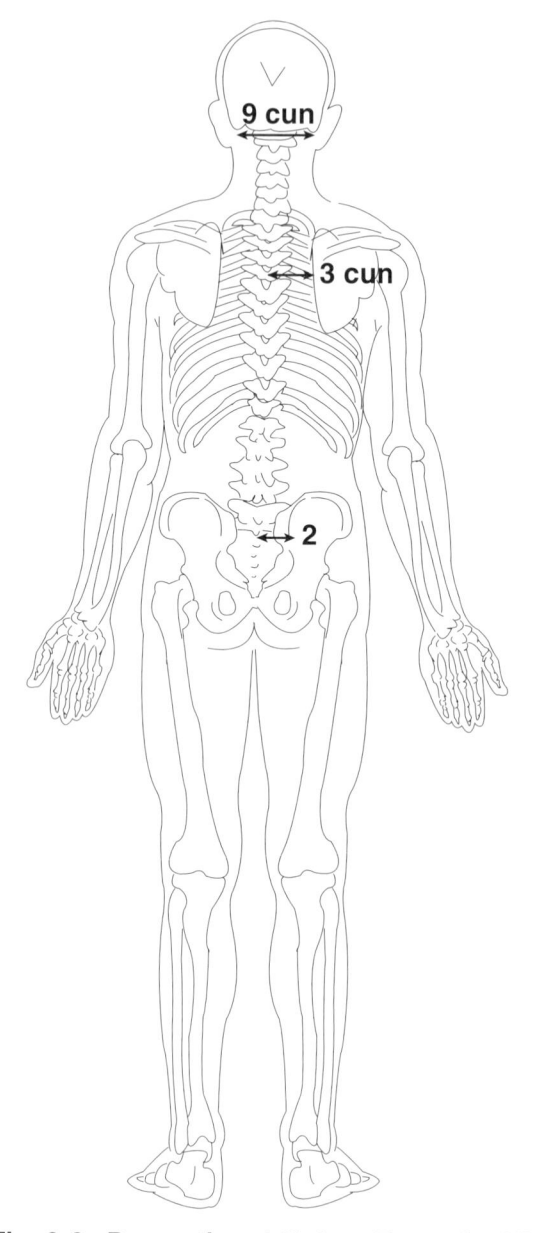

Fig. 8-3. Proportional Units - Posterior View

Finger Measurement

The finger measurement is based on patient's finger in terms of length and width.

Measuring with Thumb

- width of thumb at distal interphalangeal joint (DIP): 1 cun

Measuring with Middle Finger

- distance between distal interphalangeal joint (DIP) and proximal interphalangeal joint (PIP): 1 cun

Measuring with Fingers

- therapist is to adjust fingers with patient's fingers
- if therapist's fingers are equivalent to patient's fingers in size, measurement is based at PIP level
- if patient's fingers are smaller than therapist's fingers, measurement is based at therapist's DIP level
- if patient's fingers are larger than therapist's fingers, measurement is based at therapist's metacarpal joint (MCP) level
- 2 finger breadth: 1.5 cun
- 3 finger breadth: 2 cun
- 4 finger breadth: 3 cun

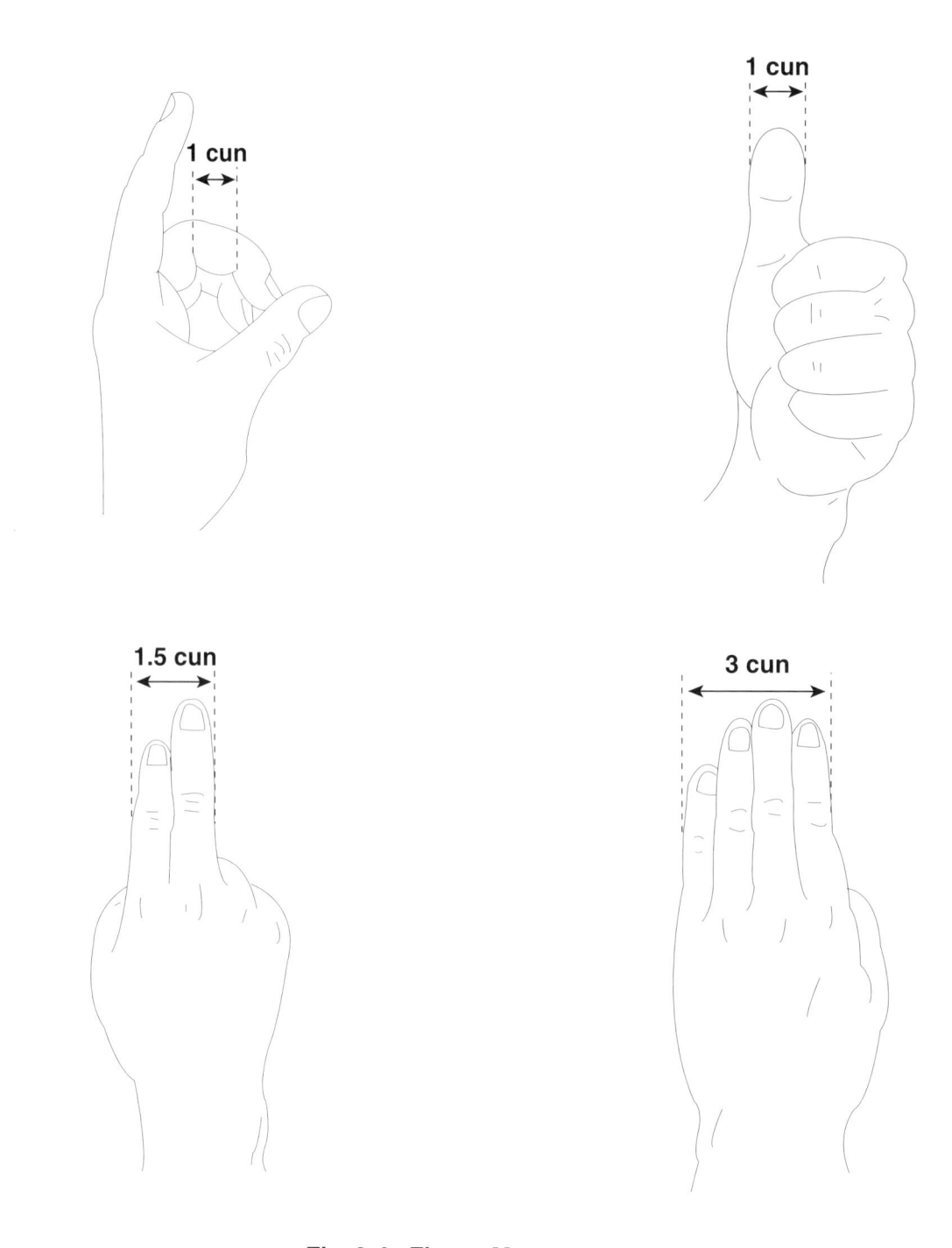

Fig. 8-4. Finger Measurements

Needle Insertion

The technique of inserting the acupuncture needle into the acupuncture point has been made much easier with the plastic guiding tube. Once the needle is percutaneous, simple rotations will help the needle to be properly placed within the acupuncture point.

After the acupuncture needle is inserted into the human body, the needle can be either manually manipulated or electrically stimulated. Electrical stimulation has only been used within the past fifty years. For most of its long history, acupuncture has been performed without electrical stimulation. In short, electrical stimulation is not a necessity aspect of acupuncture therapy. I seldom use electrical stimulation: manual stimulation is simple, easy, comfortable and, in some ways, more effective.

For manual stimulation, the acupuncture needle is manipulated by the therapist's fingers. The movements of the needle are basically of two kinds: rotatory and vertical. Another way of manipulating the needle is flipping, which gives the needle some vibration without actual movements.

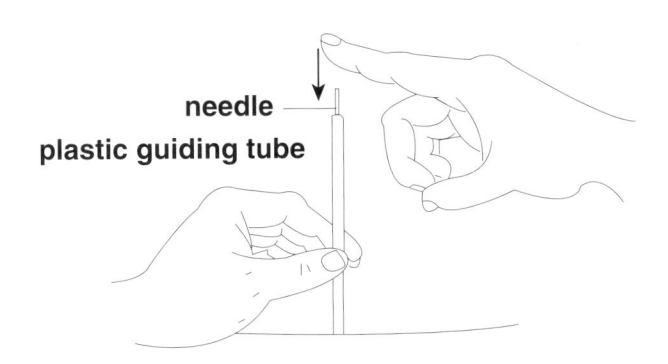

Fig. 8-5. Needle Insertion

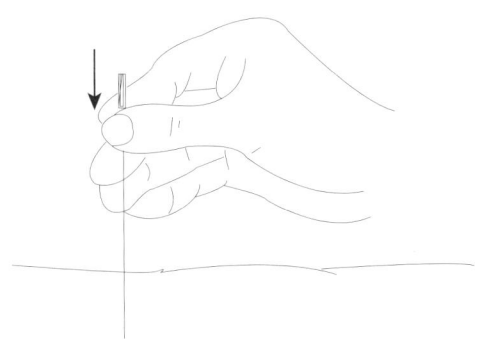

Fig. 8-6. Downward Vertical Movement of Needle

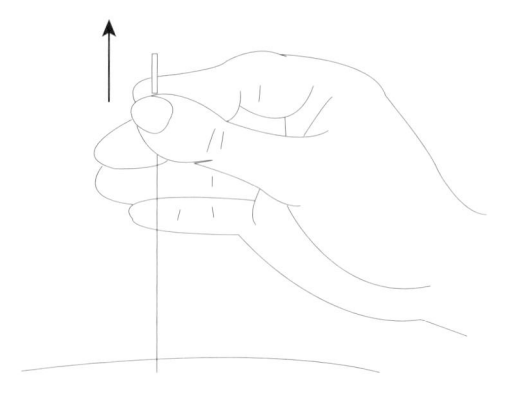

Fig. 8-7. Upward Vertical Movement of Needle

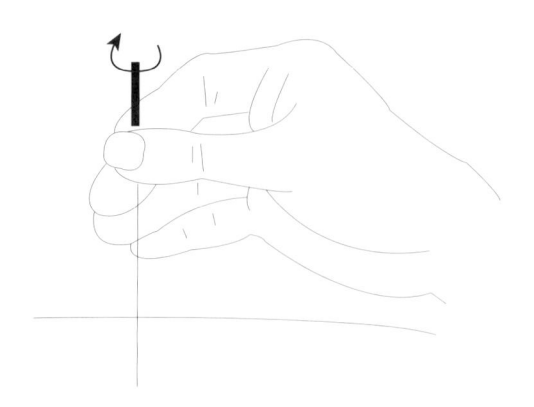

Fig. 8-8. Clockwise Rotation of Needle

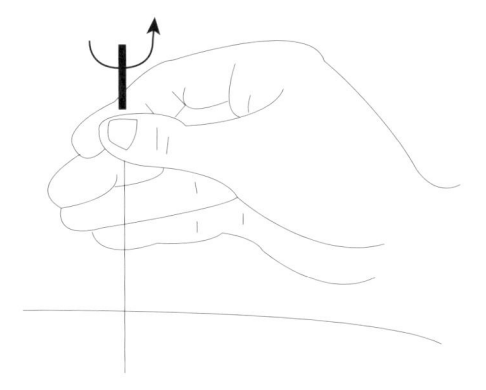

Fig. 8-9. Counter-clockwise Rotation of Needle

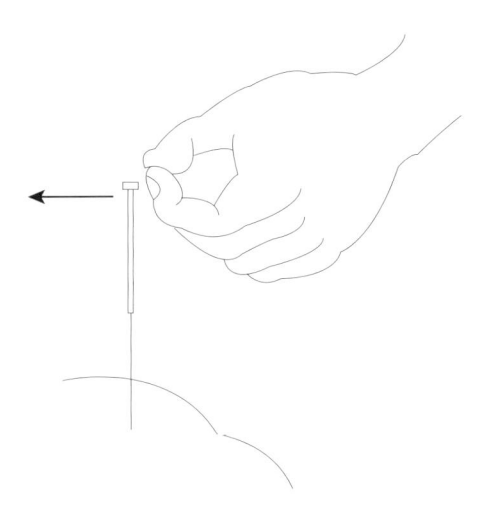

Fig. 8-10. Flipping of the Needle with Fingers

Manual Stimulation of the Needle

I divide the types of manual stimulation into three grades in terms of strength of stimulation:

---

1. Strong Stimulation

- strong stimulation done with vertical movement of needle in a pegging fashion
- strong stimulation used in some crisis situations, such as doing GV 26 for vasosyncope or vasovagal syncope of comatose patients

---

2. Moderate Stimulation

- moderate stimulation done with rotatory movements of needle
- clockwise rotation stronger than counter-clockwise rotation
- moderate stimulation used for general analgesic and anti-inflammatory purposes

---

3. Weak Stimulation

- weak stimulation done with flipping of needle with fingers – no actual movement of needle, but only some vibration
- weak stimulation used for normalization of autonomic nervous functions, as well as regenerative purposes

Electrical Stimulation of the Needle

For electrical stimulation, the acupuncture needles are connected with current through an electrical stimulator. The frequencies most commonly used are 0.6, 4, 10, 15, 50, 60, 80, 100 or 200 Hz. Experimental results have shown that low frequencies (4 Hz) may release endorphins and cortisol, while high frequencies may release serotonin for pain relief.

EA	ELECTROACUPUNCTURE
S	SENSORY RECEPTOR
N	INTER NEURON
e	ENKEPHALINERGIC NEURON
E	ENDORPHIN (-ENDORPHIN or DYNOPHIN)
NA	NORADRENALINE
H	HYPOTHALMUS
P	PITUITARY
PAG	PERIAQUEDUCTAL GRAY
RN	RAPHE NUCLEUS
RMC	RETICULAR MEGNOCELLAR NUCLEUS
DLF	DORSOLATERAL FUNICULUS

◁── STIMULATION

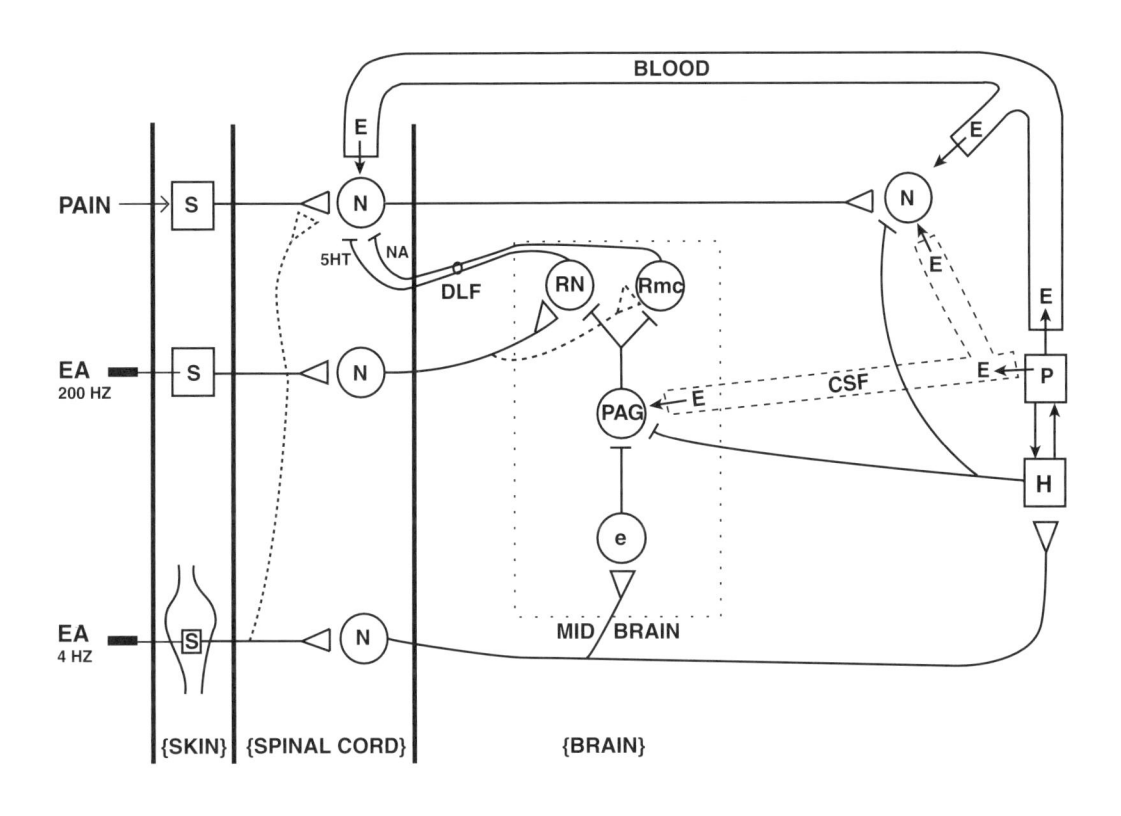

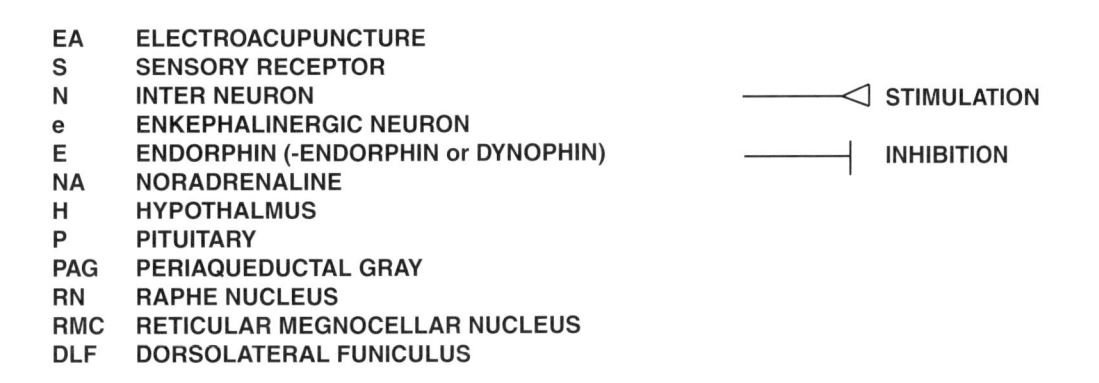

──┤ INHIBITION

Fig. 8-11. Mechanism of Elecroacupuncture Analgesia
(Cheng, R. - 1981 Ph.D. Thesis)

However, acupuncture therapy can also be effective without any manual stimulation or electrical stimulation of the needle at all.

Duration of Treatment

In dealing with pain, I have observed that in many cases some of the pain of my patients can be relieved by having the acupuncture needle inserted and removed immediately. In fact, in some instances, my patients are able to obtain substantial pain relief after having a treatment for less than one minute. However, the duration of the acupuncture treatment typically depends on the particular therapeutic goal. Consistent with my clinical experience, the following list outlines the appropriate duration for various types of treatments:

Table 8-2

Therapeutic Goal	Duration of Treatment
neurogenic pain	10 – 20 minutes
musculo-skeletal pain	1 – 10 minutes
musculo-skeletal inflammation	10 – 20 minutes
regeneration of soft tissues	30 minutes or more
normalization of autonomic dysfunction	20 – 30 minutes
surgical analgesia (induction time)	60 minutes or more

Generally, the duration is shorter for tonifying and longer for dispersing. Let me explain.

In Traditional Chinese Medicine, acupuncture stimulation can be divided into two modes – tonifying and dispersing. These are accomplished with different techniques but the most basic difference between the two methods is duration. In physical therapy, it is commonly observed that treatments of short duration tend to refresh the patient and treatments of longer duration relax and sedate the patient. A simple analogy is indicated by the difference between a quick shower and a long bath: a quick shower refreshes and energizes, a long bath relaxes and may sedate. Hence, short treatments are excitative and long treatments are sedative.

Needle Manipulation Technique in Traditional Chinese Medicine

Table 8-3

	Tonifying	**Dispersing**
insertion	slow-in rapid-out	rapid-in slow-out
vertical movement	heavy-in light-out	light-in heavy-out
rotatory movement	rotation to left	rotation to right
needle direction	needle follows direction of meridian	needle counters direction of meridian
duration of treatment	short	long

Chapter Nine

Neuro-Anatomical Acupuncture

During the ancient time in China, the knowledge of anatomy was very limited because dissection of a human body was considered as immoral. The concepts of the human psychological and emotional functions were believed to be controlled only by the heart. There were common expressions such as "heart opening" for happiness and "heart broken" for sadness...

This is perhaps one of the very original anatomy atlases in China. It is interesting to note that the brain is not existing; the uterus is also missing; the position of the heart is in the middle of the chest; the large intestine is on the right; the small intestine is on the left...

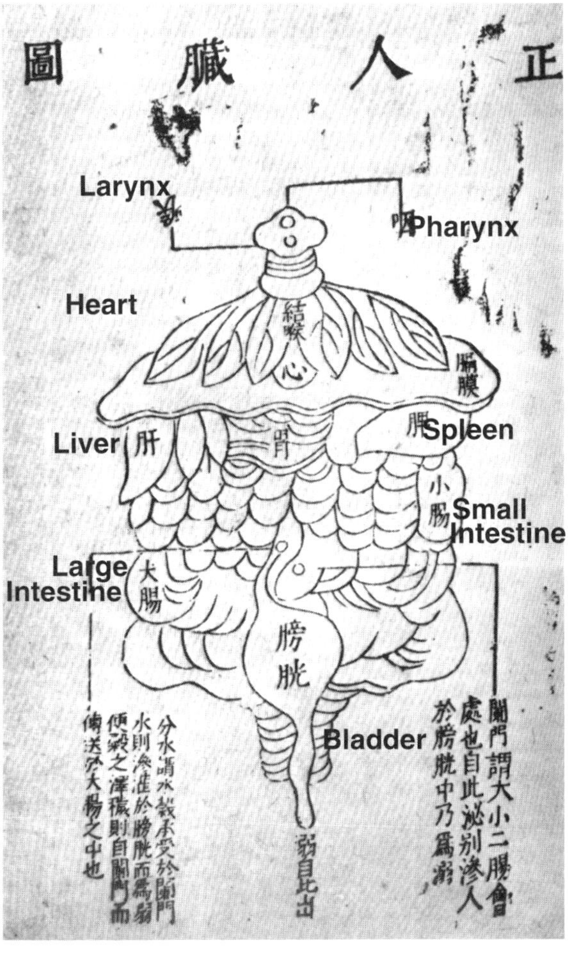

Fig. 9-1. Ancient Chinese Anatomical Drawing

The Concept of Neuro-Anatomical Acupuncture

Once the acupuncture needle is inserted into the human body, it will create physiological changes in that body. The changes may depend on which acupuncture point is used. The reception of the physical stimulus produced by the acupuncture needle relies on the nervous system. There are more than three-hundred-and-sixty basic acupuncture points along the fourteen classical meridians. The underlying anatomical structure is quite different from one acupuncture point to another. Examining the underlying anatomical structure of an individual acupuncture point may help us to understand the physiology of the acupuncture therapeutic mechanism. Acupuncture directly involves the human body and, therefore, a practitioner of acupuncture must have an adequate knowledge of human anatomy and physiology. This knowledge is requisite for both the effectiveness of the therapy and the patient's safety.

Medical professionals spend a great deal of time in university learning the anatomy, physiology and pathology of the human body. Today, for a proper diagnosis, the therapist should also utilize modern and scientifically based technologies. Effective diagnosis forms the essential basis of the modern practice of acupuncture. With respect to this fact, I have developed a different approach for the teaching and learning of a modern, scientifically based acupuncture from those approaches based solely on Traditional Chinese Medicine. I call this approach of acupuncture "neuro-anatomical acupuncture". This method makes the study and practice of acupuncture more comprehensible and effective for the medical and paramedical practitioners trained in Western medicine.

As I mentioned previously, acupuncture is essentially a form of physical therapy. The acupuncturist does not merely insert a needle into any point of the human body in order to achieve the desired therapeutic effect. The location of the needle's insertion is part of the key to the success of the therapy. Generally, in physical therapy for pain management, physical stimulus is applied to the location of the body afflicted with pain. The application of the physical stimulus is thus directly and geographically related to the pain. Physical therapy is also frequently effective in cases where stimulus is applied to tender points, trigger points or motor points.

Acupuncture points involve different anatomical structures and, in contrast to conventional physical therapy, acupuncture stimulation may be applied to a number of different locations of the body, many of which are geographically distant from the pain area of the body. However, the underlying anatomical structures of these locations are usually anatomically related to the pain area.

Twenty-eight years ago, I discovered an effective way to study acupuncture. I was in the anatomy laboratory of the University of Toronto. During that time, I had the opportunity to insert acupuncture needles into the acupuncture points of some well-dissected cadavers. By doing this, I was able to identify the underlying anatomical structures of individual acupuncture points. During this process of study, I realized that acupuncture therapy does not merely stimulate peripheral nerves but also many other surrounding anatomical structures, such as fasciae, ligaments, tendons, muscles, joints (intra-articular) and blood vessels. Furthermore, acupuncture needles can be inserted to stimulate other structures such as the neuro-plexus, the spinal nerves and the cranial nerves. In order to affect the autonomic nervous system, acupuncture needles can be inserted in places that stimulate different sympathetic nerves, parasympathetic nerves and autonomic nerve ganglions. Although the locations of the acupuncture points are not necessarily in the area of pain, they are always anatomically relevant with respect to the pain area.

The acupuncture stimulation, which is applied to the human body can be done in three different ways:

1. Direct Stimulation

The acupuncture needles can be directly inserted into different parts of the body. These can be areas of different soft tissues, peripheral nerves, spinal nerves, cranial nerves or autonomic nervous system control points. The needles are deeply inserted in order to have direct contact with particular anatomical structures. For example, a six inch needle is sometimes inserted into the buttock in order to have direct contact with the sciatic nerve. The direct stimulation of the muscle or nerve is quite similar to electromyography (EMG) but, whereas EMG is diagnostic, acupuncture can be thought of as a **therapeutic EMG**.

2. Indirect Stimulation

In some areas of the human body, acupuncture needles cannot be inserted deeply in order to have direct contact with the anatomical structures. For instance, needles must not be inserted into the brain, the lungs, the heart or the internal organs in the abdomen. Deep insertion into these areas would be very traumatic or even lethal. In order to stimulate the brain or the internal organs, acupuncture needles are often inserted into the surface of the head, the chest wall or the abdominal wall. This is effective because there is an intimate relationship between the exterior and the interior of the body. This principle – the relationship of exterior and interior – accounts for the operation of the electroencephalogram (EEG). In electroencephalography, needle electrodes are applied to the scalp and brain activities are specifically recorded. The electroencephalogram is, of course, a diagnostic procedure, yet acupuncture therapy works in a similar manner. Acupuncture applies needles to the surface of the brain, either the scalp or the face, and stimulates the brain (rather than diagnosing it). In other words, acupuncture can be thought of as a **therapeutic EEG**.

By the same token, an electrocardiogram (ECG) is used to record the activities of the heart. Again, the ECG demonstrates the specific and intimate relationship between the exterior and interior of the body. Acupuncture can be performed in a similar fashion: the acupuncture needle is inserted into the surface of the chest wall but in order to stimulate rather than diagnose the lungs and the heart. Here, acupuncture performs as a **therapeutic ECG**.

3. Projectional Stimulation

Acupuncture can be administered on a small part of the human body in order to control the other parts of the human body in a projectional fashion. Here, acupuncture needles can be applied to the external ear, the nose, the hand and the foot. These areas are considered to be microsystems within the framework of acupuncture.

It is believed that all systems of acupuncture have originated in China and are perhaps based on the medical text, "The Yellow Emperor Classic of Internal Medicine". Nevertheless, the ancient Chinese ear acupuncture points were not organized somatotopically. In the 1950's, Dr. Paul Nogier, a neurologist from Leon, France, developed a somatotopic map of the external ear, based upon the concept of the orientation of an inverted fetus. In 1960, more research work was carried out in China to verify the clinical accuracy of the Nogier's ear homunculus. This ear acupuncture is later called **auriculo-medicine**.

Nose acupuncture, hand acupuncture and **foot acupuncture** have been developed from the meridian theory in China. The significance of these acupuncture treatments is that many diseases can be treated with the use of acupuncture points which are located only in the nose, hand or foot. In the 1970's, in Korea, Tae-Woo Yoo presented **Korean hand acupuncture**, which is a more complicated and sophisticated microsystem.

Point of Stimulation

Neuro-anatomical acupuncture is an approach in acupuncture therapy based on the anatomy and physiology of the human body. As mentioned, in most of the physical therapy modalities, the stimulus is always applied to the painful site in dealing with pain. However, in acupuncture, the physical stimulus can be applied to different sites other than the pain site:

- pain site
- peripheral nerve
- neuro-plexus
- spinal nerve
- cranial nerve
- autonomic nerve points – panic switches, sympathetic switches, parasympathetic switches
- sympathetic ganglion
- indirect stimulation points – brain stimulation, chest stimulation, abdominal stimulation
- projectional acupuncture points in microsystems of ear, nose, hand and foot

Chapter Ten

Normalization of the Autonomic Nervous Dysfunction with Acupuncture

Acupuncture is known to balance the yin and yang principles of the human body. This is compatible with the idea of normalization of the sympathetic and parasympathetic dysfunctions of the human body.

Autonomic Nervous Crisis (i.e. shock)

- central:
  - ***panic switches*** in head: GV 20, GV 26
- peripheral:
  - ***panic switches*** in upper extremity: LU 11, PC 9, HT 9, LI 1, TH 1, SI 1, Shixuan (extra-meridian)
  - ***panic switches*** in lower extremity: KI 1

Autonomic Nervous Control of Head

- sympathetic: BL 2, GB 20
- parasympathetic: BL 1, ST 1, TH 17, CV 24
- control from neck: SI 17 (superior cervical sympathetic ganglion), ST 9

Autonomic Nervous Control in Neck

- sympathetic: GB 20, GV 14, SI 17 (superior cervical sympathetic ganglion), ST 10 (middle cervical sympathetic ganglion), ST 11 (inferior cervical sympathetic ganglion)
- parasympathetic: CV 22, ST 9

Autonomic Nervous Control in Upper Extremity

- major **sympathetic switches**: LI 4, LI 11
- major **parasympathetic switches**: PC 6, HT 7
- special sympathetic switches for musculo-skeletal disorders: TH 5, SI 3

Autonomic Nervous Control in Lower Extremity

- major **sympathetic switches**: LR 3, ST 36
- major **parasympathetic switches**: SP 6, BL 40
- special sympathetic switches for musculo-skeletal disorders: GB 34, BL 60

Autonomic Nervous Control in Back

- major sympathetic control: BL 23, GV 4
- major parasympathetic control: BL 32, BL 33

A neuro-anatomical approach to acupuncture – utilizing knowledge of anatomy and the biochemical mechanisms of the human body – brings about a much better understanding of acupuncture therapy. This approach allows us to understand the empirical and scientific basis of acupuncture. Traditional Chinese Medicine has given us, in acupuncture, a powerful therapeutic tool, based on thousands of years of careful observation and experience. Thanks to ongoing studies and research, perhaps many of the discoveries of Traditional Chinese Medicine will be much better understood in the near future.

Table 10-1

Acupuncture Point	Location
GV 20	on midline of head, 7 cun anterior to posterior hair margin, midpoint on a line connecting apex of two auricles
GV 26	superior to midpoint of philtrum
LU 11	on radial side of thumb, 0.1 cun to corner of nail
PC 9	at tip of middle finger
HT 9	on radial side of little finger, 0.1 cun to corner of nail
LI 1	on radial side of index finger, 0.1 cun to corner of nail
TH 1	on ulnar side of 4th finger, 0.1 cun to corner of nail
SI 1	on ulnar side of little finger, 0.1 cun to corner of nail
Shixuan	at tip of all fingers
KI 1	on sole of foot between 2nd and 3rd metatarsal bones, proximal to MTT joint
GB 20	in depression between upper ends of sternocleidomastoid and trapezius muscles
BL 1	0.1 cun superior to medial canthus
BL 2	on medial end of eyebrow, on supra-orbital notch
ST 1	between eyeball and midpoint of infra-orbital ridge
CV 24	midpoint of mental labial fossa
TH 17	posterior to lobule of ear, between mandible and mastoid process
SI 17	posterior to angle of mandible, anterior to sternocleidomastoid muscle

Acupuncture Point	Location
ST 9	level with tip of thyroid cartilage, at anterior border of sternocleidomastoid muscle
GV 14	midline of spine between C 7 and T 1 spinous processes
ST 10	midpoint between ST 9 and ST 11 at anterior border of sternocleidomastoid muscle
ST 11	midpoint between sternal head and clavicular head of sternocleidomastoid muscle, immediately superior to clavicle
CV 22	on anterior midline, at center of suprasternal fossa
LI 4	between 1st and 2nd metacarpal bone at midpoint of 2nd metacarpal bone
LI 11	at lateral end of elbow crease, midpoint between lateral epicondyle and biceps aponeurosis in cubital fossa
PC 6	2 cun proximal to palmar wrist crease between tendons of palmary longus and flexor carpi radialis
HT 7	on wrist crease, on radial side of flexor carpi ulnaris tendon
TH 5	2 cun proximal to dorsal wrist crease between ulna and radius
LR 3	between 1st and 2nd toes, midpoint at 2nd metatarsal
SI 3	on ulnar side of metacarpal bone, proximal to MCP joint
ST 36	3 cun inferior to lower margin of patella, 1 cun lateral to crest of tibia
SP 6	3 cun superior to tip of medial malleolus on posterior border of tibia

Acupuncture Point	Location
BL 40	on popliteal crease midpoint of popliteal fossa
GB 34	in depression anterior and inferior to head of fibula
BL 60	in depression between lateral malleolus and Achilles tendon
BL 23	1.5 cun from midline of spine between L 2 and L 3
GV 4	midline of spine between L 2 and L 3 spinous processes
BL 32	1 cun from midline of spine in 2nd sacral foramen
BL 33	1 cun from midline of spine in 3rd sacral foramen

Chapter Eleven

The Therapeutic Strategies of Neuro-Anatomical Acupuncture

The therapeutic outcome of acupuncture treatment for musculo-skeletal disorders depends on the following elements:

- accurate diagnosis
- good selection of acupuncture points
- precision of needle insertion and placement
- appropriate stimulus variables
  - manual stimulation: different techniques and duration
  - electrical stimulation: intensity, frequency and duration

With accurate diagnosis, good acupuncture point selection, precision of needle insertion and placement, appropriate stimulus variables, the therapeutic result of acupuncture is often seen ***instantaneously***.

Repeated Examination

Careful clinical examination is necessary to derive an accurate diagnosis. It is important to examine the patient immediately before and immediately after the acupuncture treatment. Failing to do so, the therapist may risk missing information valuable for the therapy. Anytime the therapeutic result is not instantaneous or satisfactory, it is probable one or more of the four critical elements outlined above has not been correctly performed. In this case, all four elements should be re-examined and suitable adjustments made in order to achieve a better result for the next treatment.

One Needle Approach

Selection of acupuncture points can be done in different ways. A one acupuncture needle approach is often best for the first treatment of a new patient. When a large number of acupuncture needles are inserted at the same time, the therapist may have difficulty discerning which needle is producing a good result. The specificity of the one needle approach can help verify the therapist's diagnosis. Clearly this approach is the most beneficial for a new patient because it allows the therapist accurately and specifically to pinpoint both the problem and the best treatment program.

Multiple Acupuncture Points Program

A multiple acupuncture points program uses a combination of different acupuncture points. Initially, the acupuncture point in the area of pain can be used. The peripheral nerve points or spinal nerve points can also be added at the same time. These points should be anatomically related to the disorder. For example, in treating supraspinatus tendinitis, the suprascapular nerve points are the points of choice since the supraspinatus muscle is innervated by the suprascapular nerve. By the same token, the C 5 spinal nerve points should also be used for this condition, as they represent the relevant spinal segment.

Autonomic nervous acupuncture points can also be incorporated into the treatment program. In fact, when a patient presents with a problem involving very intense pain, the physical examination might be so difficult that an accurate diagnosis cannot be made right away. In this case, it is very helpful to make the autonomic nervous acupuncture points the first line of approach. This allows the therapist to reduce, at a general level, the severity of pain the patient is experiencing. When the severity of pain is alleviated, re-examination of the patient will allow the therapist to obtain a more specific and accurate diagnosis. Accordingly, the patient can then be treated through the use of other acupuncture points – points in the area of pain, as well as the peripheral nerve points and the spinal nerve points.

Needle Insertion and Placement

The precision of needle insertion and placement is critically important. The location of acupuncture points by finger measurement is a very convenient method. However, at times, due to individual anatomical variation, this method may not be completely accurate. Therefore, other landmarks should also be taken into consideration, such as those indicated by muscle, tendon and bone.

The correct direction of needle insertion is also very important. Furthermore, for direct stimulation, the right depth of needle insertion is also significant.

Manual Stimulation Versus Electrical Stimulation

Stimulation variables refer to different manual stimulation techniques and different intensity, frequency and duration. As previously mentioned, electrical stimulation is not necessary for acupuncture therapy – acupuncture was successfully performed without electric current in China for approximately three thousand years. Electric current has only been available within the last couple of hundred years. Electro-acupuncture has been used within the past fifty years. Through my acupuncture experience of more than forty years, I have not found significant difference in the result between these two methods.

How Important is the De-Qi Sensation?

The De-Qi sensation is a sensation that the patients experience during acupuncture when needles are inserted. Usually, the description of this sensation is vague, but patients have described it as follows: "numbness, tingling, aching-feeling, warmth, skin-crawling". In Traditional Chinese Medicine, it is believed that without this sensation a favorable result may not be achieved.

Using the appropriate landmarks and inserting the acupuncture needle precisely, I have noted that even if the patient does not have any De-Qi sensation a good therapeutic result can still be achieved. In fact, because finer needles are being used today, patients may hardly feel the needles at all. Hence, the patients do not necessarily experience pain or any other sensation as the needle is inserted. Therefore, the De-Qi sensation is not an absolute indication of the outcome of the treatment.

Acupuncture Therapeutic Program

If, during the first treatment, the patient experiences an instantaneous and positive therapeutic result, the next question is how to organize an effective therapy program. The program should be very intensive. In fact, I believe that it is extremely important to see and treat a new patient on a daily or even twice daily basis for at least two to three consecutive days. By doing this, the following advantages are obtained:

- better pain control (acupuncture's effectiveness is cumulative)

- greater accuracy in diagnosis (close observation allows therapist to check and recheck initial diagnosis and make appropriate changes in selection of acupuncture points)

The intensive approach dramatically increases the success rate of therapy.

Naturally, therapeutic goals of a treatment program should be set according to the clinical problem encountered (for example, pain and inflammation). The frequency of the treatments can then be established in a regime such that treatment frequency will gradually be reduced, for example, moving from daily treatments to treatments of three times weekly, then two times weekly and then once weekly. The overall duration of the program must be decided on an individual basis according to the patient's progress.

Acupuncture with Other Associated Therapies

When dealing with musculo-skeletal disorders, it is very advantageous to engage in other treatment modalities, either at the same time or immediately after the acupuncture treatment. Treatments involving any of the following modalities work well in concert with acupuncture:

- manipulation
- mobilization
- exercises

Acupuncture needles must, however, be inserted distal to the areas where manipulation, mobilization or exercises are being performed. The needles should not interfere with the movements involved in such treatments. The result of combining acupuncture with these treatments is often spectacular if not miraculous. Projectional acupuncture, particularly ear acupuncture, can also be used with these other treatments modalities.

Holistic Approach

When dealing with chronic disorders, attention must be paid to any other physical dysfunctions present in the body. Common problems, such as bowel and bladder dysfunctions, fatigue and sleeping disorders must also be attended to. Furthermore, the patient's pain problem may also be influenced by any concomitant disease such as systemic rheumatological disorders (rheumatoid arthritis, lupus erythematosus, etc.), hypertension, diabetes mellitus and thyroid dysfunctions. Most of these diseases can be alleviated by means of acupuncture. The patient's emotional status should also be taken into consideration: depression or anxiety can adversely affect the outcome of treatment. A holistic approach should always be kept in mind.

Touch-Up Technique

Upon finishing each acupuncture treatment, the therapist should re-examine the patient in order to see if any pain is still present. Most patients report an immediate reduction of pain after a treatment session. However, if there is still pain present, the patient may now be able to localize the area of pain more precisely. Accordingly, another minute of acupuncture applied to the specific area of pain may completely eliminate it. In fact, every effort should be taken to make the patient if not totally pain-free then as painless as possible following each treatment. To repeat, acupuncture's effectiveness is cumulative: the touch-up approach enhances the cumulative effectiveness of acupuncture treatment in order to produce the best overall reduction of pain.

Repeated Performance

I have noticed that acupuncture seems to be more effective if the treatment is repeated with the same acupuncture point or points. The repetition is within one session of the treatment with very short intervals:

- treatment for one minute followed by interval of one minute
- repeat same treatment for one minute followed by interval of one minute
- repeat same treatment for one minute followed by interval of one minute…

Very obvious improvement is usually noticed immediately.

Chapter Twelve

Possible Hazards and Complications of Acupuncture

Syncope

It is not uncommon for certain patients to develop a light-headed sensation during or after an acupuncture treatment. This sensation may last for a few minutes or a couple of hours. Occasionally, some patients faint after insertion of an acupuncture needle. This is recognized as vasosyncope or vasovagal syncope. In this event, the inserted acupuncture needles should be removed immediately. The patient should then be put in the Trendelenburg position (lying in a supine position, legs raised). In order to revitalize the patient, insert another acupuncture needle in the acupuncture point, GV 26. Usually, there will be a prompt response to this treatment.

It is always important to inquire into the patient's history of fainting. To help prevent fainting, all new patients should be placed in a lying position during treatment.

This complication is usually easily resolved.

Seizure

On rare occasions, a patient may have a seizure during an acupuncture treatment. In the past forty years, I have only seen a few such cases among my acupuncture patients. Most of these patients had a past history of seizure and recovered spontaneously. Although rare, a patient's seizure may range from petit mal to grand mal.

Hemorrhage

Occasionally, minor bruising occurs during or immediately following an acupuncture treatment, particularly if the treated area has an abundant distribution of superficial veins. Insertion of an acupuncture needle around the eye may, on rare occasions, result in a "black eye". The bruised area should vanish completely within a couple of days.

At other times, a hematoma may be produced at an acupuncture point where an artery has been injured.

Prior to acupuncture therapy, the patient should be asked if they have a history of hemophilia or other blood disorders. Special attention should also be paid to those who are on anticoagulant medications.

Perforation of Viscus

Major danger or even death could result if an acupuncture needle is inserted into a vital organ, such as the brain, the heart, the lungs and the abdominal organs. It is critically important that all acupuncture therapists should be familiar with the landmarks of the vital organs. The therapist must be aware of all acupuncture points through which the acupuncture needle could reach a vital organ.

Statistics indicate that **pneumothorax** is more commonly reported than any other incidences. Therefore, extra attention must be paid to the outlines of the heart, lungs and pleura. (see Fig. 12-1 and Fig. 12-2)

Infection

It is extremely rare for a patient treated with proper precautions to develop bacterial skin infection from acupuncture therapy. The patient's skin should be prepared for the acupuncture needle with seventy percent alcohol solution. The acupuncture therapist should wash his hands prior to the acupuncture treatment. Precautions should also be taken regarding viral infections such as hepatitis, HIV, etc. In fact, the acupuncture treatment can be performed by the therapist wearing sterilized surgical gloves and using forceps if some patient is especially prone to infection.

Broken Needle

The acupuncture needle is made of fine steel and the shaft of the acupuncture needle is not easily broken. However, the junction between the shaft and the handle is the weakest part of the needle. It is advisable that the needle should not be fully inserted. Thus, if there were any breakage, the needle could be easily pulled out with a pair of forceps.

Masking of Other Co-Existing Diseases

Practicing acupuncture should not be any different than practicing any other form of medicine. An accurate diagnosis is extremely important. Every effort should be made to avoid masking serious organic conditions, such as heart disease, malignancy, etc.

Electro-Acupuncture Hazards

In electro-acupuncture, if excessive intensity and frequency are used, skin tattooing or burns (minimal) can occur.

Precaution should be taken when applying the needles of electro-acupuncture to areas near the heart. Excessive intensity and frequency could interfere with cardiac function, particularly if the patient has a cardiac pacemaker.

Pregnancy

Acupuncture treatment can be contra-indicated during pregnancy, particularly during the first trimester because some acupuncture points have strong autonomic nervous functional influence and could potentially cause contraction of the uterus. Nevertheless, I have treated a large number of pregnant patients during their first trimester for hyperemesis, using acupuncture point PC 6, with no adverse effect at all. However, the acupuncture points in the major spinal autonomic nervous centers must definitely be avoided. This includes all the points in the back and abdomen below T 10. The peripheral autonomic nervous points in the extremities should also be avoided.

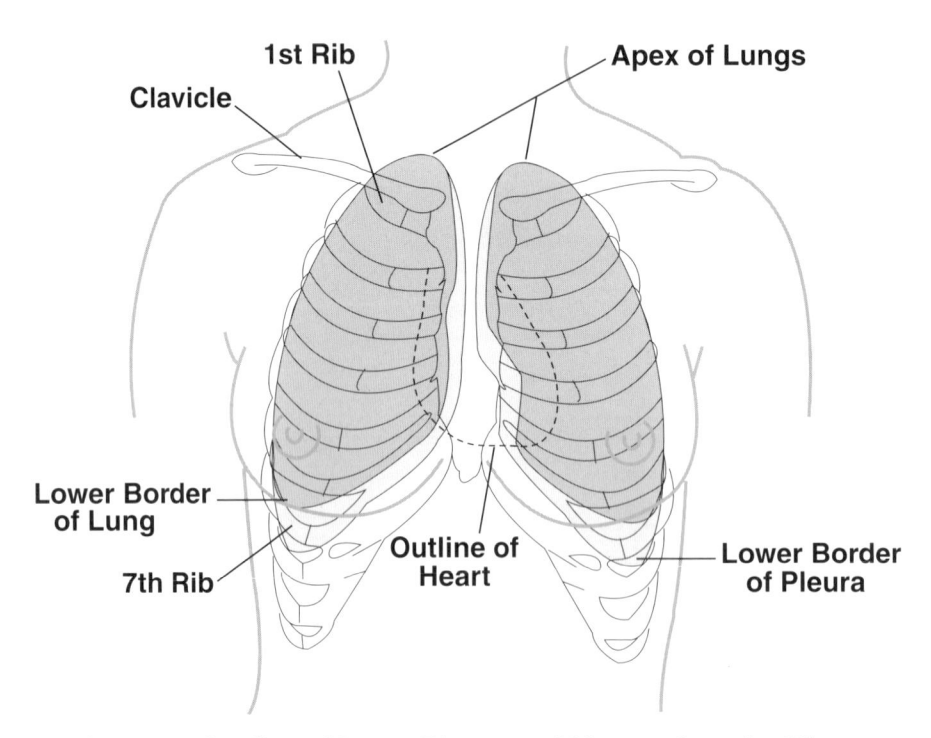

Fig. 12-1. Outline of Lung, Pleura and Heart - Anterior View

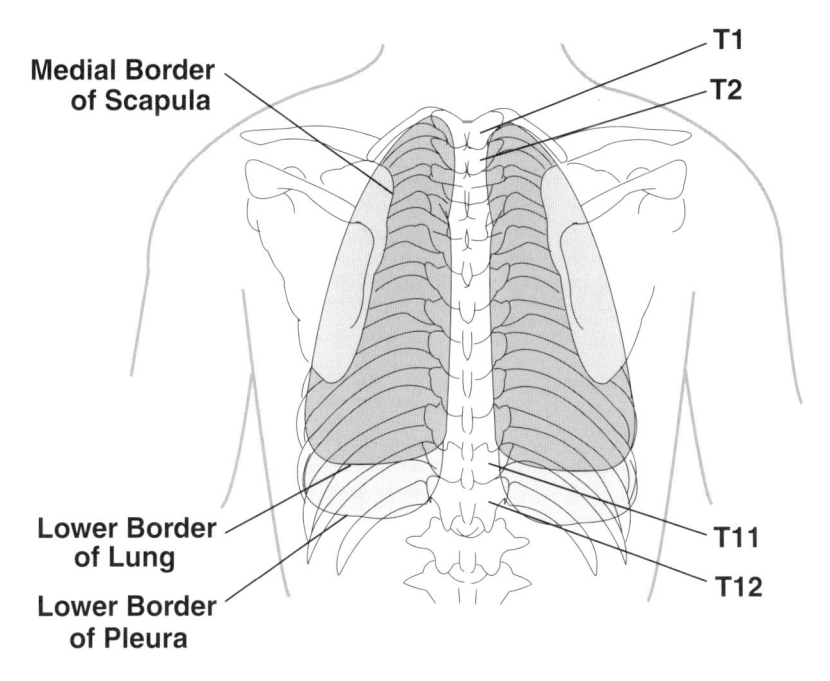

Fig. 12-2. Outline of Lung and Pleura - Posterior View

Chapter Thirteen

The Neck

Acupuncture Meridians and Points in the Neck

There are four meridians crossing the **_posterior aspect_** of the neck:

Table 13-1

Meridian	Acupuncture Point	Location
Governing Meridian (GV)	GV 14	midline of spine between C 7 and T 1 spinous processes
	GV 15	midline of spine between C 1 posterior tubercle and C 2 spinous process
	GV 16	midline of spine between C 1 posterior tubercle and occipital bone
Urinary Bladder Meridian (BL)	BL 10	1.3 cun lateral to GV 15
Gallbladder Meridian (GB)	GB 12	posterior and inferior to mastoid process
	GB 20	in depression between upper ends of sternocleidomastoid and trapezius muscles
Small Intestine Meridian (SI)	SI 15	2 cun lateral to GV 14

There are five meridians crossing the ***anterolateral aspect*** of the neck:

Table 13-2

Meridian	Acupuncture Point	Location
Conception Meridian (CV)	CV 22	on anterior midline, at center of suprasternal fossa
	CV 23	on anterior midline, immediately superior to hyoid bone
Stomach Meridian (ST)	ST 9	level with tip of thyroid cartilage, at anterior border of sternocleidomastoid muscle
	ST 10	midpoint between ST 9 and ST 11, at anterior border of sternocleidomastoid muscle
	ST 11	midpoint between sternal head and clavicular head of sternocleidomastoid muscle, immediately superior to clavicle
	ST 12	at midpoint of supraclavicular fossa, 4 cun lateral to midline of chest
Large Intestine Meridian (LI)	LI 17	level with ST 10, posterior to sternocleidomastoid muscle
	LI 18	level with ST 9, midpoint between bellies of sternocleidomastoid muscle
Small Intestine Meridian (SI)	SI 16	0.5 cun posterior to LI 18
	SI 17	posterior to angle of mandible, anterior to sternocleidomastoid muscle
Triple Heater Meridian (TH)	TH 16	level with angle of mandible, posterior to sternocleidomastoid muscle
	TH 17	posterior to lobule of ear, between mandible and mastoid process

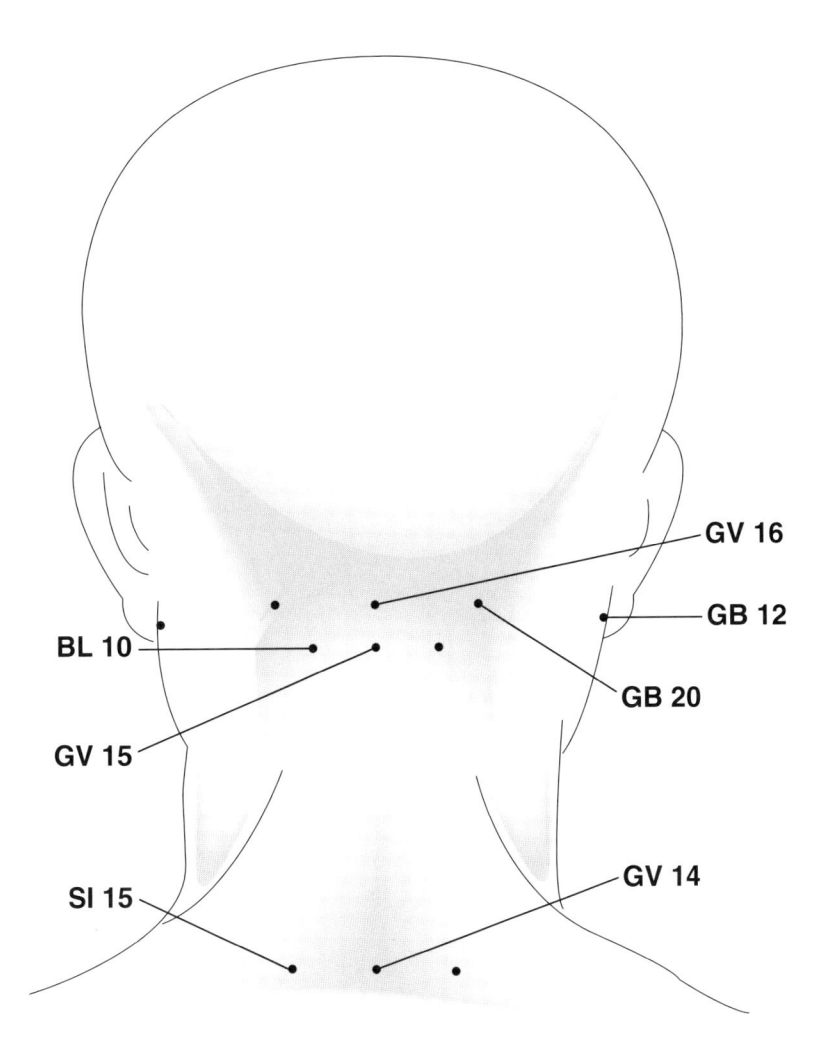

Fig. 13-1. Acupuncture Points in the Neck
- Posterior Surface View

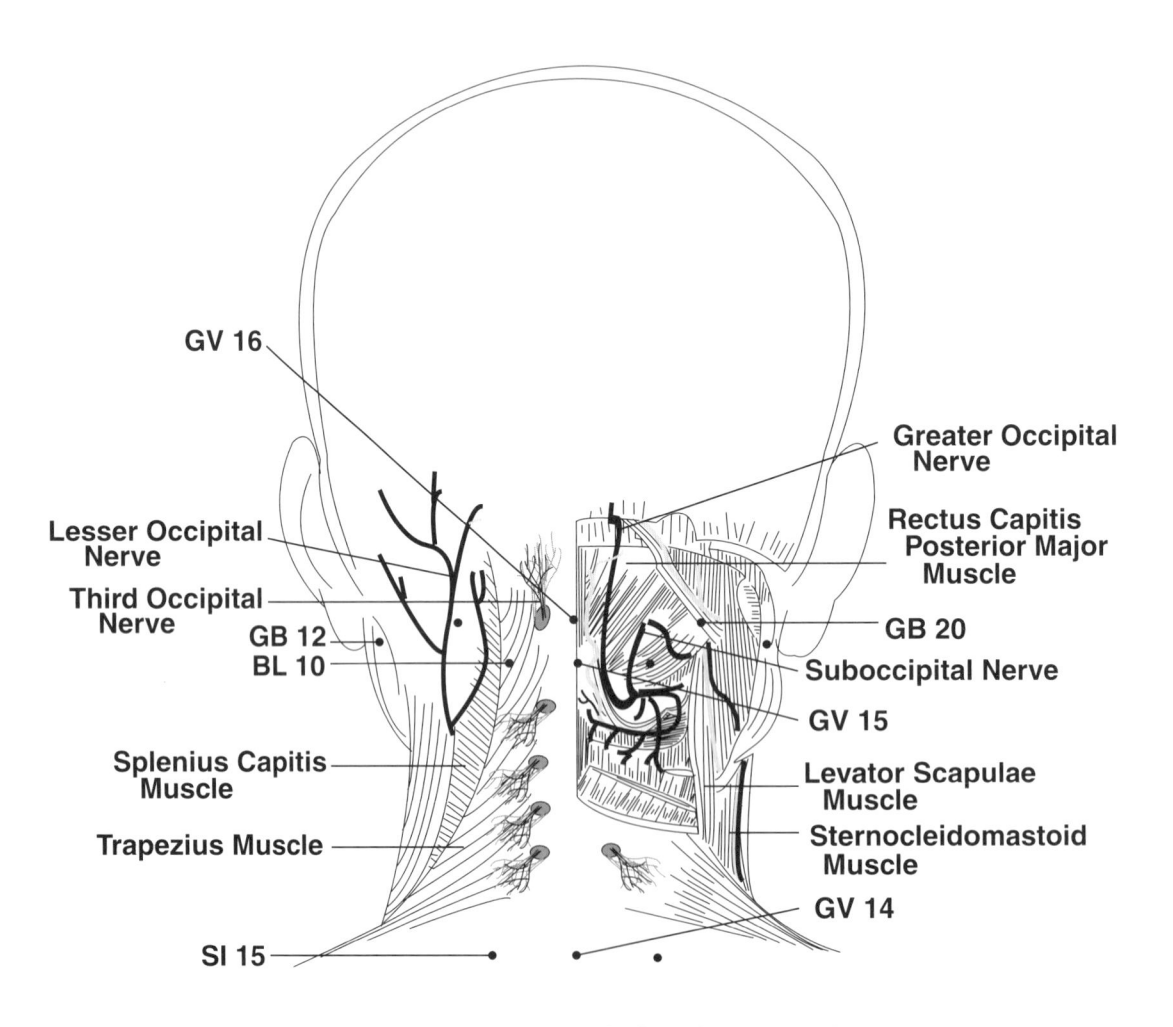

Fig. 13-2. Acupuncture Points in the Neck
- Posterior Deeper View

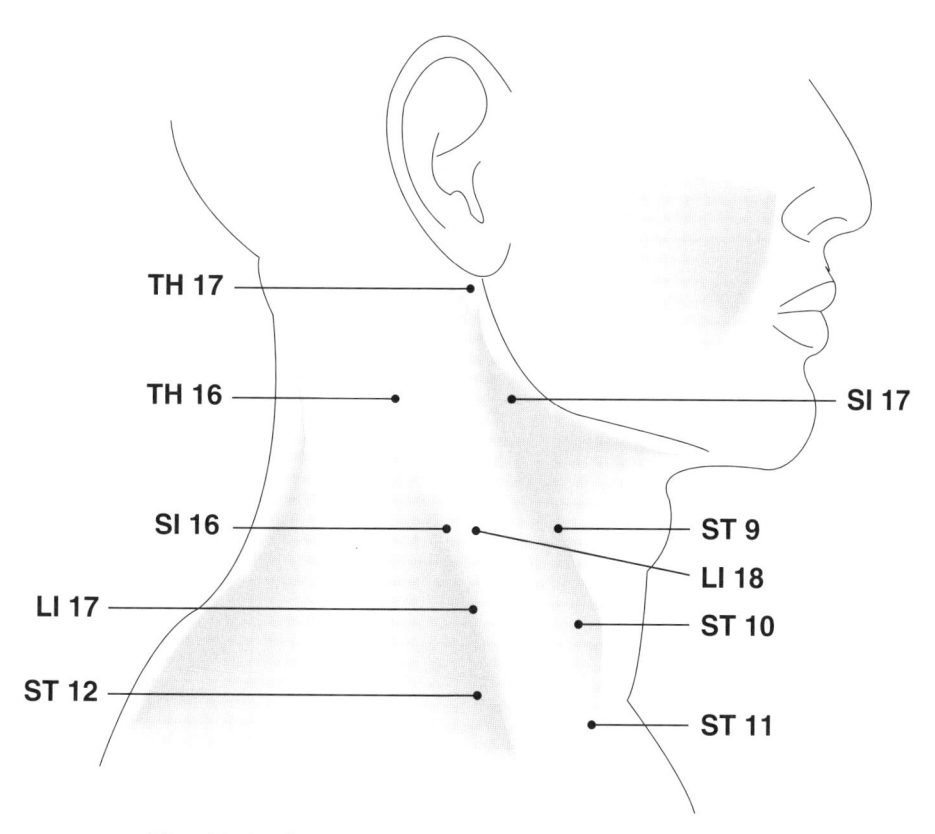

Fig. 13-3. Acupuncture Points in the Neck
- Lateral Surface View

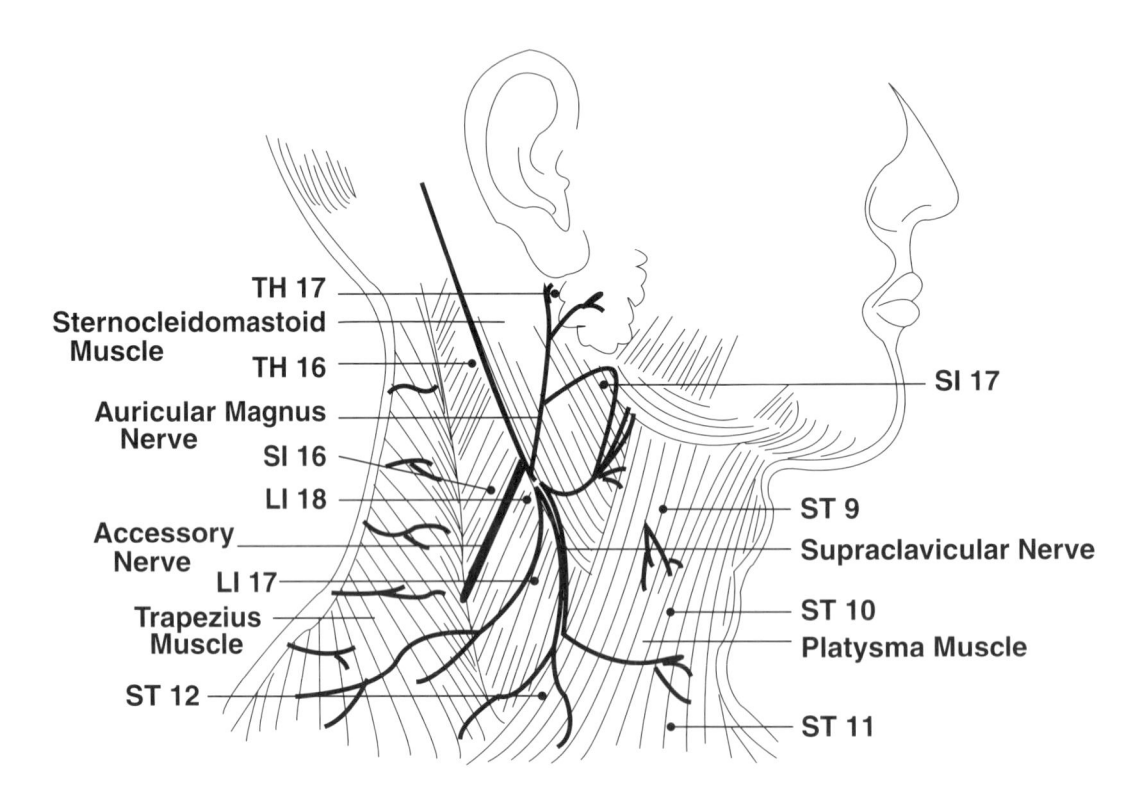

Fig. 13-4. Acupuncture Points in the Neck
- Lateral Superficial View

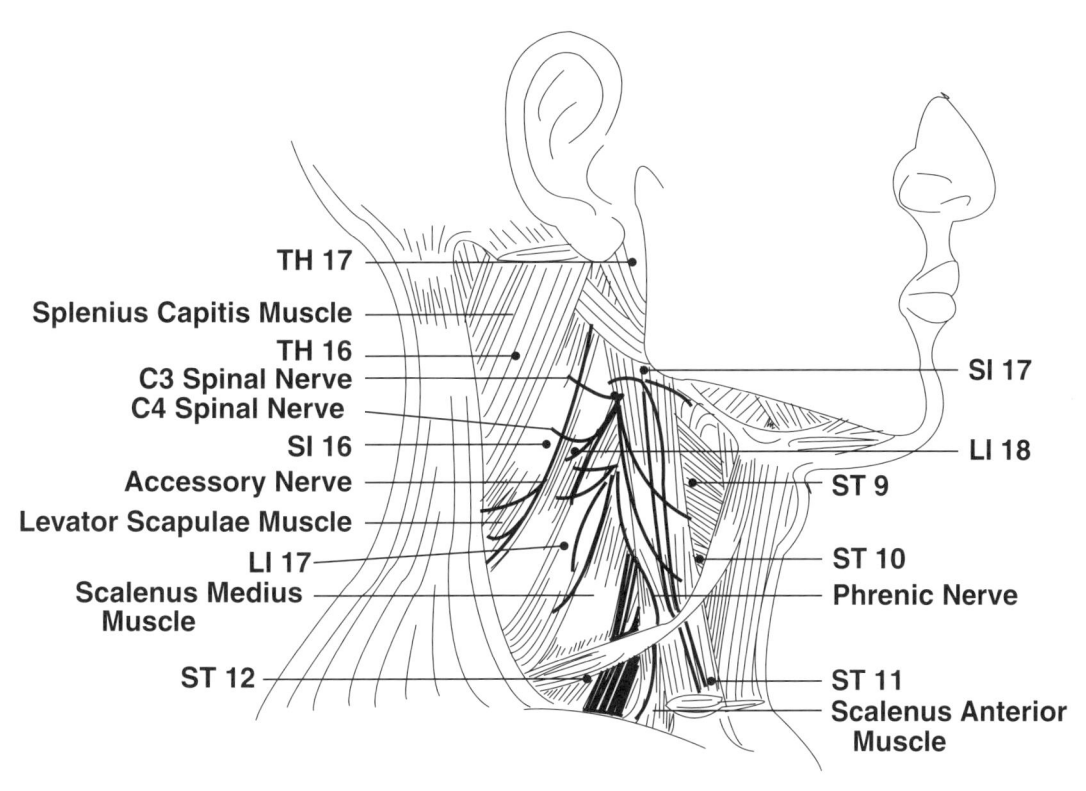

Fig. 13-5. Acupuncture Points in the Neck
- Lateral Middle View

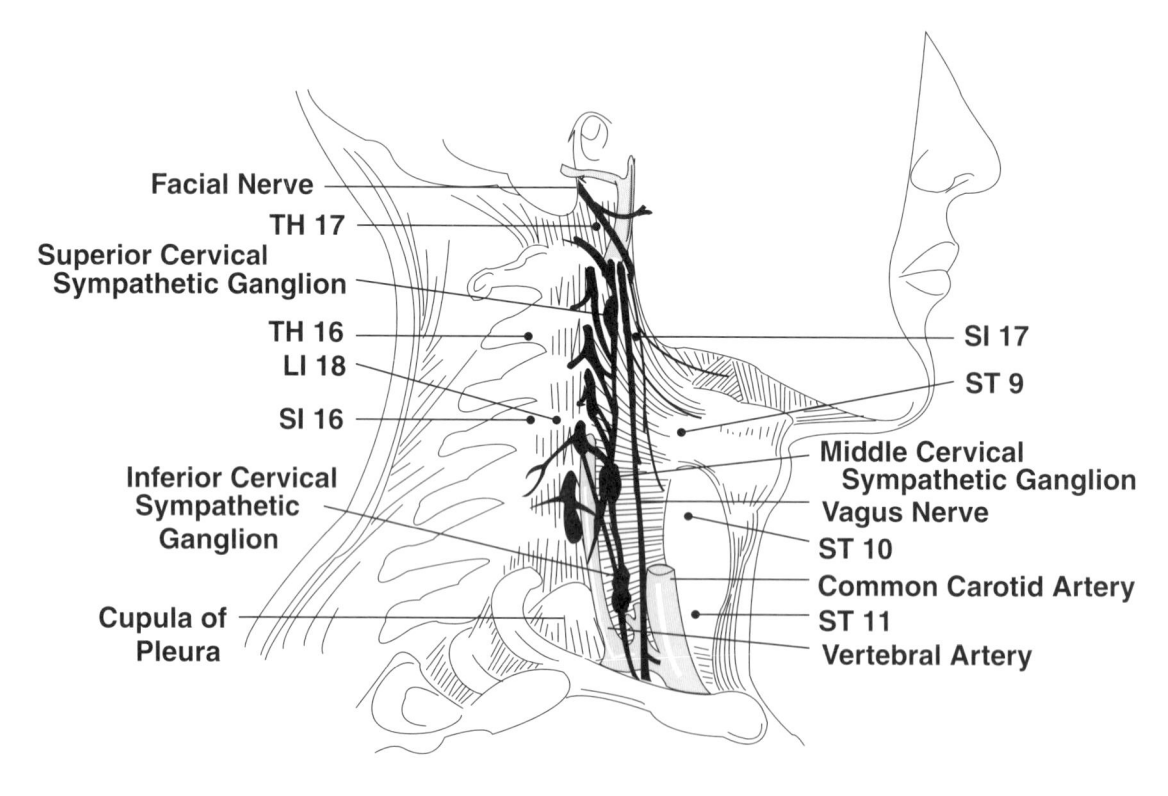

Fig. 13-6. Acupuncture Points in the Neck
- Lateral Deep View

Extra-Meridian Points

Table 13-3

Acupuncture Point	Location
Extra GV point (interspinal)	following design of GV 14 and GV 15, add acupuncture point on midline of spine between any two spinous processes at all spinal segments
Extra BL point (paraspinal 1.3 cun)	following design of BL 10, add acupuncture point on urinary bladder meridian line, 1.3 cun lateral to midline of spine at all spinal segments
Huatuojiaji point (paraspinal 0.5 cun)	0.5 cun lateral to midline of spine at all spinal segments
Facet Joint point (paraspinal 1.0 cun)	1 cun lateral to midline of spine at all spinal segments
Cervical Spinal Nerve point (lateral-spinal)	extra-meridian point on lateral aspect of neck, posterior to posterior border of sternocleidomastoid muscle at all spinal segments
Ding Chuan	1 cun lateral to GV 14

GV 16
GV 15

Extra GV
Points

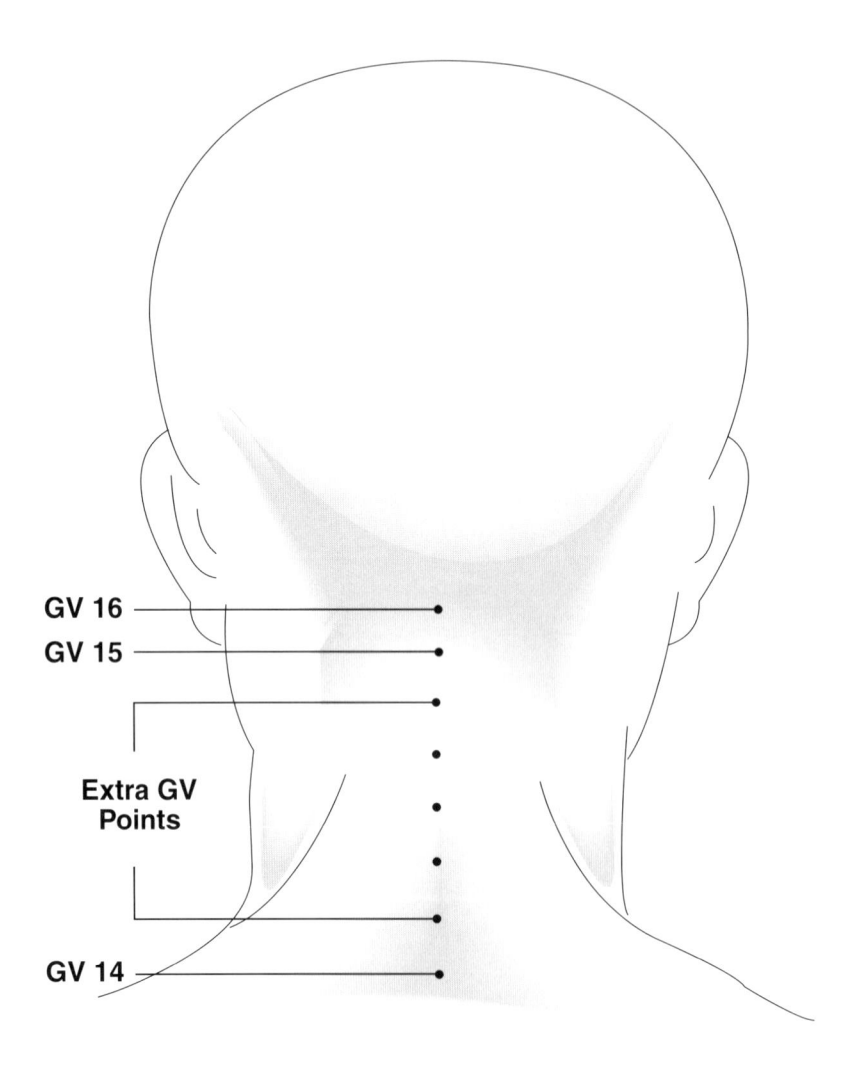

GV 14

Fig. 13-7. Extra-Meridian Points in the Neck
- Extra GV Points

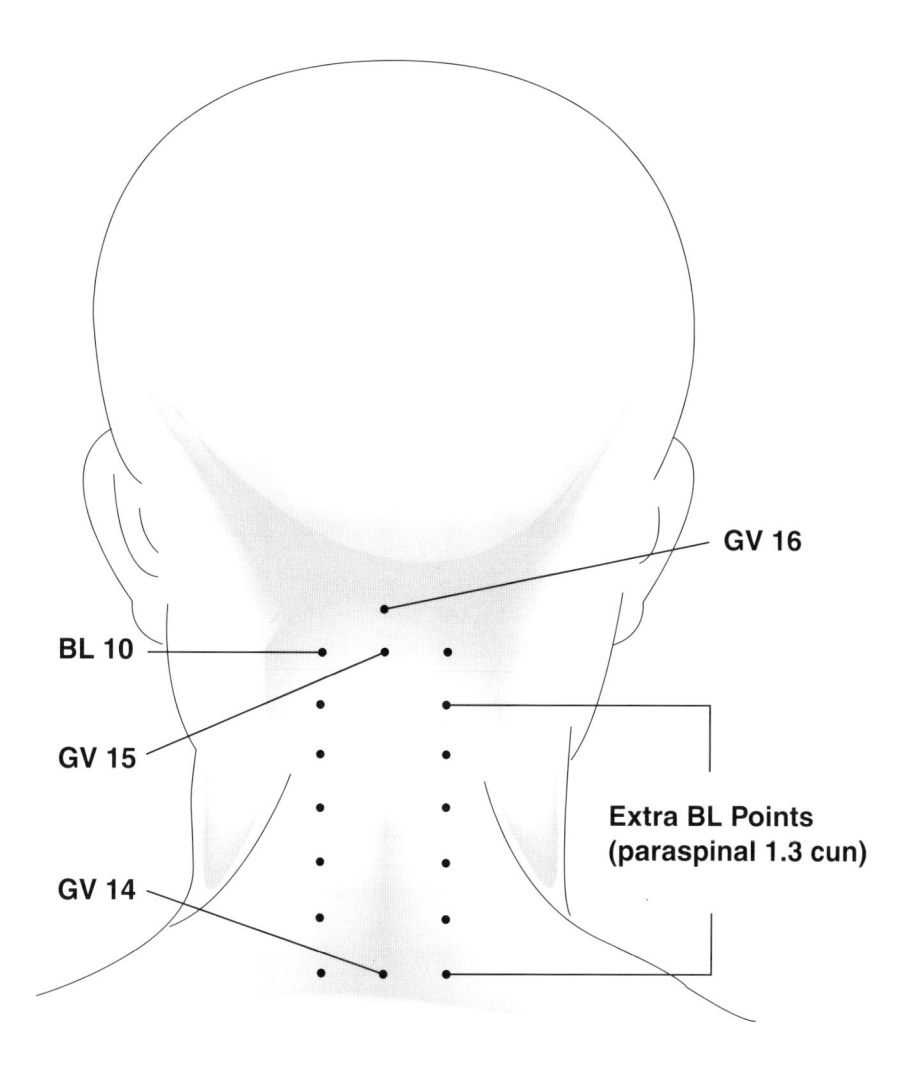

Fig. 13-8. Extra-Meridian Points in the Neck
- Extra BL Points

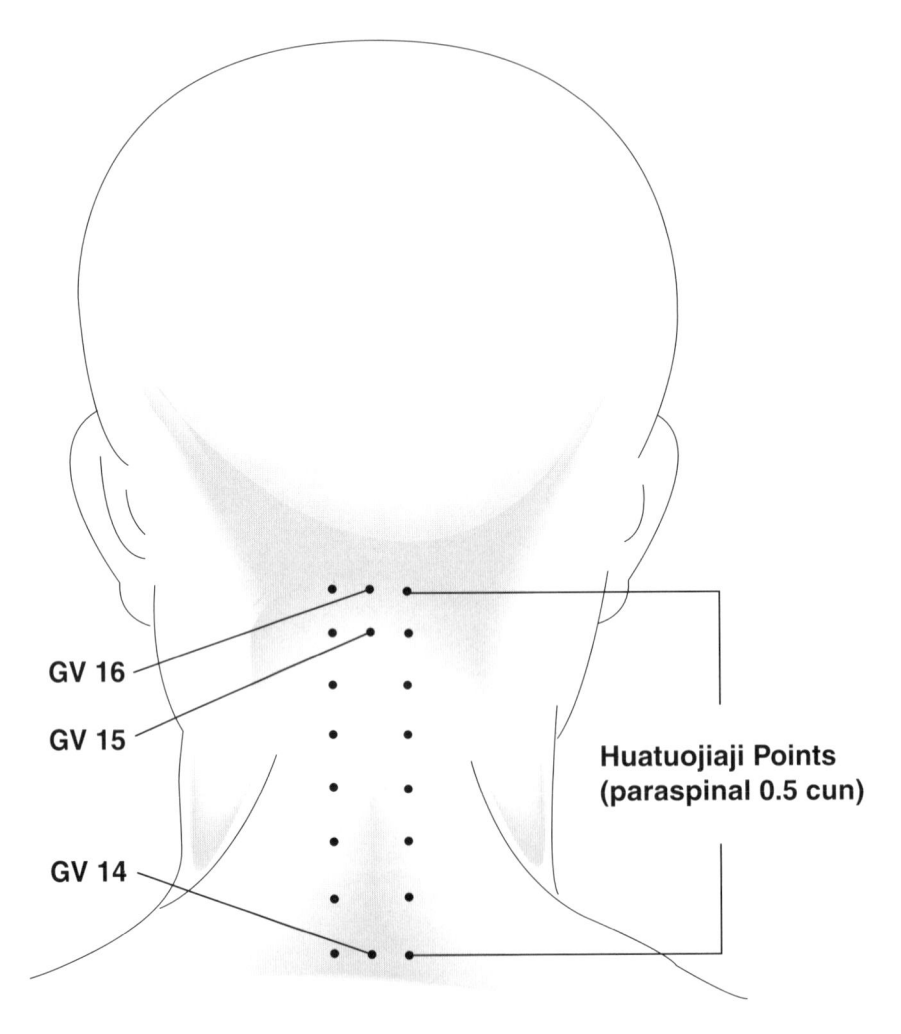

**Fig. 13-9. Extra-Meridian Points in the Neck
 - Huatuojiaji Points**

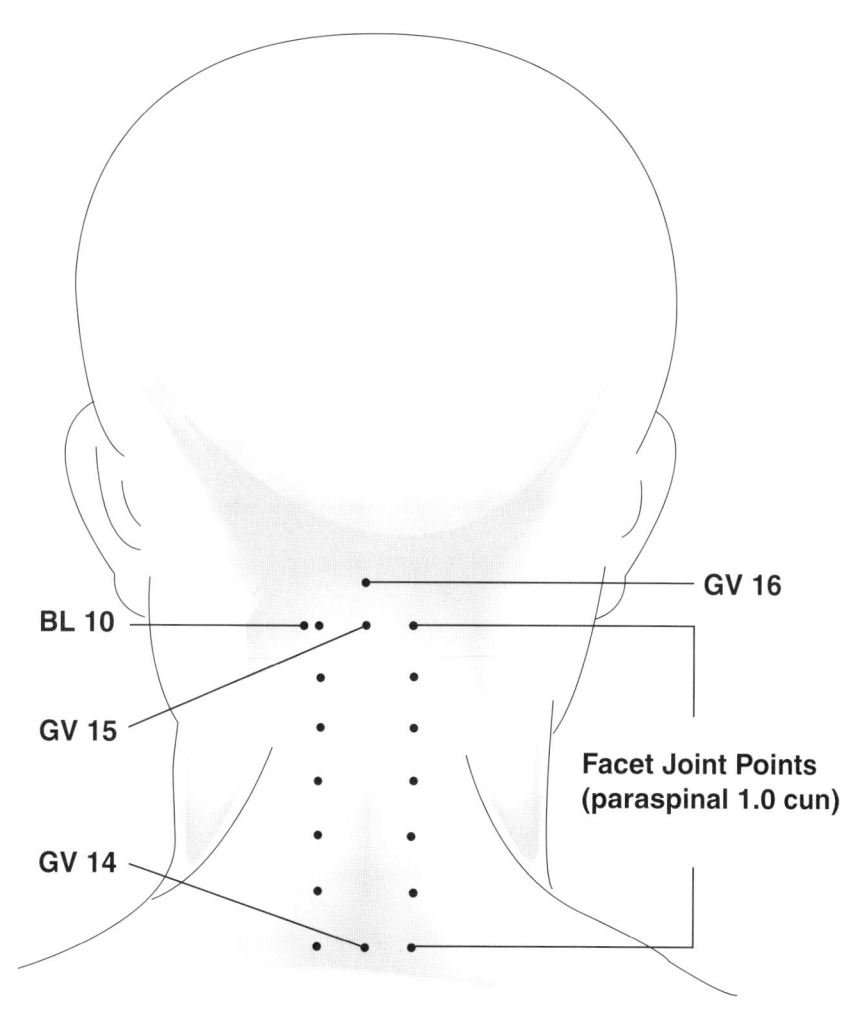

Fig. 13-10. Extra-Meridian Points in the Neck
- Facet Joint Points

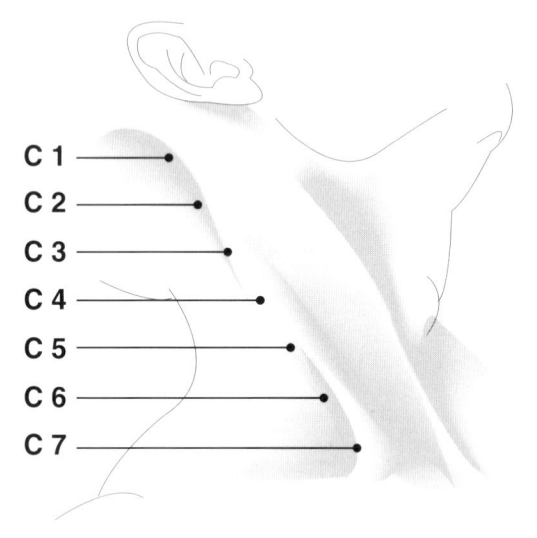

C 1: Inferior to the Mastoid Process
C 2: Superior to the Mandibular Angle
C 3: Hyoid Bone
C 4: Upper Margin of the Thyroid Cartilage
C 5: Lower Margin of the Thyroid Cartilage
C 6: First Cricoid Ring
C 7: Superior to the Clavicle

Fig. 13-11. Extra-Meridian Points in the Neck
 - Cervical Spinal Nerve Points (Surface View)

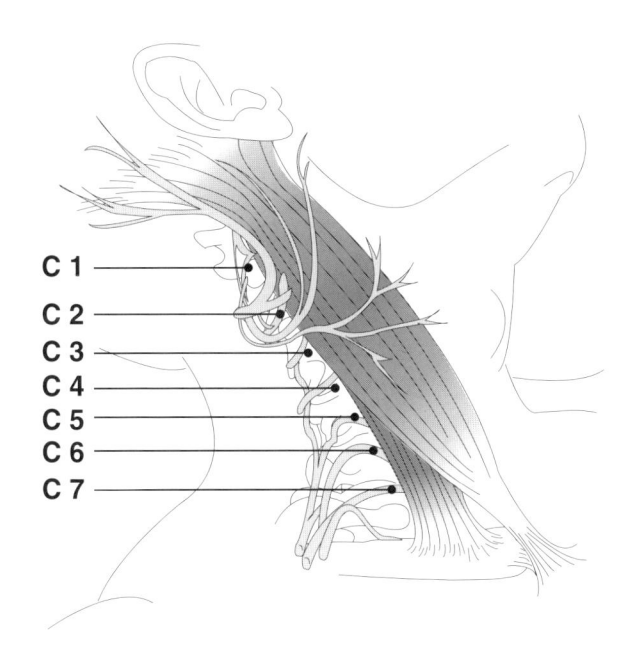

Fig. 13-12. Extra-Meridian Points in the Neck
    - Cervical Spinal Nerve Points (Deeper View)

Nerve Stimulation in the Neck

Table 13-4

	Name of Nerve	Acupuncture Point
Cranial Nerve	7th cranial nerve (facial nerve)	TH 17
	9th cranial nerve (glossopharyngeal nerve)	CV 23, ST 9, SI 17
	10th cranial nerve (vagus nerve)	ST 9, ST 10, ST 11, CV 22
	11th cranial nerve (accessory nerve)	GB 20, LI 18
	12th cranial nerve (hypoglossal nerve)	CV 23
Spinal Nerve	medial branch of posterior primary ramus	GV 14, GV 15, GV 16, Extra GV points
	lateral branch of posterior primary ramus	BL 10, Extra BL points
	anterior primary ramus	C 1 to C 7 spinal nerve points (extra-meridian)
	sinu-vertebral nerve*	C 1 to C 7 Huatuojiaji points (extra-meridian)
Peripheral Nerve	suboccipital nerve	GB 12, GV 16
	greater occipital nerve	BL 10
	third occipital nerve	Huatuojiaji point at C 1, C 2 level
	lesser occipital nerve	GB 20, SI 16
	greater auricular nerve	GB 20, SI 16, TH 17
	dorsal scapular nerve	SI 15
	phrenic nerve	LI 17
Neuro-Plexus	cervical plexus	spinal nerve point at C 4 level
	brachial plexus	ST 12, LU 2

Name of Nerve		Acupuncture Point
Cervical Sympathetic Ganglia	superior cervical sympathetic ganglion	SI 17
	middle cervical sympathetic ganglion	ST 10
	inferior cervical sympathetic ganglion (plus stellate ganglion)	ST 11

*Sinu-Vertebral Nerve

The sinu-vertebral nerve, a recurrent branch of each spinal nerve, is reflected back through the intervertebral foramen to supply the articular connective tissues, periosteum, meninges and vascular structures. The nerve originates from:

1) anterior primary divisions of the spinal nerves,

2) gray ramus communicans of the sympathetic system.

It supplies dura mater, posterior longitudinal ligament and the annulus of intervertebral disc.

Cervical Muscles

Table 13-5

Muscle	Action	Peripheral Nerve	Spinal Segment	Acupuncture Point
Sternocleido-mastoid	bends head and neck toward shoulder; rotates head toward opposite side; both sides act together to flex neck and head	accessory nerve, C 2, C 3 spinal nerves	C 2, C 3	GB 20, BL 10, LI 18, GV 15
Trapezius	raises shoulder; extends head; bends head toward shoulder; rotates scapula	accessory nerve, C 2 - C 4 spinal nerves	C 2 - C 4	GB 20, BL 10, LI 18, GV 15
Semispinalis Capititis	extends head and bends it laterally	C 1 - C 5 (posterior rami)	C 1 - C 8	GV 15, GV 16, BL 10, Extra GV points C 1 - C 5 spinal segments; Extra BL points C 1 - C 5 spinal segments
Longus Coli	flexes neck	C 2 - C 6 spinal nerves	C 2 - C 6	C 2 - C 6 Spinal Nerve points
Longus Capitis	flexes head and rotates it toward same side	C 1 - C 4 spinal nerves	C 1 - C 3	C 1 - C 4 Spinal Nerve points

Muscle	Action	Peripheral Nerve	Spinal Segment	Acupuncture Point
Rectus Capitis Anterior	flexes head and rotates it toward same side	C 1 spinal nerve	C 1, C 2	GV 16, GB 12,
Rectus Capitis Lateralis	bends head to side	C 1 spinal nerve	C 1	GV 16, GB 12, C 1 Spinal Nerve point
Rectus Capitis Posterior Major	extends and rotates head	suboccipital nerve	C 1	GV 16, GB 12, Extra BL point at C 1 level
Rectus Capitis Posterior Minor	extends head	suboccipital nerve	C 1	GV 16, GB 12, Extra BL point at C 1 level
Obliquus Capitis Inferior	rotates head	suboccipital nerve	C 1	GV 16, GB 12, Extra BL point at C 1 level
Obliquus Capitis Superior	extends head	suboccipital nerve	C 1	GV 16, GB 12, Extra BL point at C 1 level
Levator Scapulae	draws scapula upward	C 3, C 4 spinal nerves	C 3, C 4	SI 13, TH 15, GB 21, Spinal Nerve points C 3, C 4
Anterior Scalene	raises 1st rib; bends neck to same side	C 5 - C 7 spinal nerves	C 5 - C 7	Spinal Nerve points C 5 - C 7
Middle Scalene	raises 1st and 2nd ribs; bends neck to same side	C 4 - C 8 spinal nerves	C 4 - C 8	Spinal Nerve points C 4 - C 7
Posterior Scalene	raises 1st and 2nd ribs; bends neck to same side	C 7 spinal nerves	C 7	Spinal Nerve point C 7

Clinical Application

Degenerative Disc Disease (Osteoarthritis)

- highest incidence at C 5 - C 6 level
- higher cervical levels may result in occipital neuralgia
- involvement of spinal nerves may result in radicular pain and paresthesia
- GV 14, GB 20, GV 15, GV 16 for occipital headache
- Extra GV point (interspinal) for the respective spinal segment
- Extra BL point (paraspinal) for the respective spinal segment
- BL 10 for the spinal segment C 1 - C 2

Cervical Radicular Pain

- proximal pain with distal paresthesia
- brachial plexus points (ST 12, LU 2, HT 1) control proximal pain
- LI 4 (radial nerve), PC 6 (median nerve), HT 7 (ulnar nerve) reduce distal paresthesia
- treat underlying pathology in neck (rule-out discogenic disorders)

Cervical Nerve Roots and Symptoms

Spinal Segments	Radicular Symptoms
C 3 (C 2 - C 3)	pain and numbness in posterior cervical area around mastoid process and pinna of ear
C 4 (C 3 - C 4)	pain and numbness in posterior cervical area radiating along levator scapula and occasionally to anterior chest
C 5 (C 4 - C 5)	pain radiating from lateral cervical area to shoulder top; numbness over middle of deltoid
C 6 (C 5 - C 6)	pain radiating down lateral side of arm and forearm often to thumb and index finger
C 7 (C 6 - C 7)	pain radiating to middle of forearm and middle three fingers of hand
C 8 (C 7 - T 1)	pain radiating to forearm and ring and little fingers with numbness, rarely extends above wrist

Rheumatoid Arthritis

- uncommon for rheumatoid arthritis to affect cervical spine only
- watch for Atlanto-axial subluxation
- BL 10 for the spinal segment C 1 - C 2
- GV 15 also controls this level
- Extra GV point (interspinal) for the other respective spinal segment
- Extra BL point (paraspinal) for the other respective spinal segment
- rheumatoid arthritis is an auto-immune disease, add immune mechanism points: LI 4, ST 36, BL 23, SP 10, SP 6

| **Immune Mechanism Points** |

LI 4, ST 36   –   to increase secretion of ACTH (via hypothalamus – pituitary complex)

BL 23   –   to facilitate production of endogenous cortico-steroids

SP 10, SP 6   –   to promote immune function (via venous and lymphatic system)

Ligamentous Strain of Cervical Spine

- Huatuojiaji point for the respective spinal segment
- GV 15, BL 10 for the C 1 - C 2 spinal segment
- GV 16 for Atlanto-occipital level
- GV 14 for C 7 level
- Extra GV point (interspinal) for the respective spinal segment
- Extra BL point (paraspinal) for the respective spinal segment

Musculo-Tendinous Strain

- acupuncture points for individual cervical muscles (see Table 13-5)

Cervical Facet Syndrome

- Cervical Facet Joint point (paraspinal 1 cun) for the respective spinal segment
- Spinal Nerve points for the respective spinal segment
- better result if acupuncture treatment followed with cervical mobilization, manipulation or exercises

Occipital Neuralgia

- may result from traumatic, degenerative, infectious, neoplastic or aneurysmal disease of upper neck region
- BL 10 for greater occipital nerve
- GB 20, SI 16 for lesser occipital nerve
- Huatuojiaji point for third occipital nerve at C 1 level

Whiplash Injury

- usually hyperextension and hyperflexion mechanism
- most commonly, soft tissues around Atlanto-occipital joints and Atlanto-axial joints, posterior ligaments and zygapophyseal joints
- very acute stage:
  - GV 26 in face
  - LI 4, SI 3 in upper limb
  - GB 34, LR 3 in lower extremity
- SI 17 (superior cervical sympathetic ganglion) to normalize sympathetic dysfunctions in neck and head
- chronic stage:
  - GB 12, GV 15, GV 16 to reduce inflammation as well as to regenerate injured tissues
  - Huatuojiaji points for the cervical spinal segment

Torticollis

- spasmodic torticollis may result from trauma, infection or subluxation of an unilateral zygapophyseal joint
- tendency for neck to twist to one side
- GB 20, LI 18 to control affected sternocleidomastoid muscle
- also C 2, C 3 spinal nerve points of affected side
- spastic torticollis may be caused by lesion in central nervous system (MRI may rule this out)

Thoracic Outlet Syndrome

- compression symptoms of neurovascular bundle (subclavian artery and brachial plexus)
- Cervical Spinal Nerve points at C 3 - C 4 spinal segment for scalenus muscles, particularly anterior scalene muscle
- Brachial Plexus points ST 12, LU 2, HT 1
- distal points HT 7 for referring pain and paresthesia in upper extremity

Fibromyalgia

- widespread musculo-skeletal pain of neck, shoulders and upper limbs
- fatigue, headache, waking unrefreshed, forgetfulness, poor concentration and depression
- multiple hyperalgesic tender spots
- GB 20, GV 14, GV 21, SI 15 to alleviate tender spots
- LI 4, LI 11 to control wide-spread inflammation and promote energy
- GB 24.5, GV 20 for depression and forgetfulness
- brain stimulation for pain facilitates patient's own pain relief mechanism (see Table 7-2)
- also treat concomitant disease in concomitant fibromyalgia (i.e. rheumatoid arthritis, hypothyroidism, hormonal disturbance...)

Cervical Sympathetic Symptoms

- vague and indefinite symptoms include migratory headache, dizziness, blurred vision, tinnitus or dysphagia
- possible compression of vertebral artery
- GB 20, GV 14, SI 17 to normalize sympathetic dysfunctions
- watch out for Horner's syndrome (unilateral enophthalmos, ptosis, myosis and flushing of face

Cervical Discogenic Paresis or Paralysis

- Cervical Spinal Nerve points at the respective spinal segments according to myotomes of muscles involved
- ST 12, LU 2, HT 1 for stimulation of brachial plexus
- strengthening exercises during acupuncture treatment

Chapter Fourteen

The Back and the Perineum

Acupuncture Meridians and Points in the Back and the Perineum

There are six meridians crossing the back:

Table 14-1

Meridian	Acupuncture Point	Location
Governing Meridian (GV)	GV 14	midline of spine between C 7 and T 1 spinous processes
	GV 13	midline of spine between T 1 and T 2 spinous processes
	GV 12	midline of spine between T 3 and T 4 spinous processes
	GV 11	midline of spine between T 5 and T 6 spinous processes
	GV 10	midline of spine between T 6 and T 7 spinous processes
	GV 9	midline of spine between T 7 and T 8 spinous processes
	GV 8	midline of spine between T 9 and T 10 spinous processes
	GV 7	midline of spine between T 10 and T 11 spinous processes
	GV 6	midline of spine between T 11 and T 12 spinous processes
	GV 5	midline of spine between L 1 and L 2 spinous processes

Meridian	Acupuncture Point	Location
Governing Meridian (GV)	GV 4	midline of spine between L 2 and L 3 spinous processes
	GV 3	midline of spine between L 4 and L 5 spinous processes
	GV 2	midpoint at hiatus sacralis
	GV 1	midpoint between coccyx and anus
Urinary Bladder Meridian (BL)	BL 11	1.5 cun from midline of spine between T 1 and T 2
	BL 12	1.5 cun from midline of spine between T 2 and T 3
	BL 13	1.5 cun from midline of spine between T 3 and T 4
	BL 14	1.5 cun from midline of spine between T 4 and T 5
	BL 15	1.5 cun from midline of spine between T 5 and T 6
	BL 16	1.5 cun from midline of spine between T 6 and T 7
	BL 17	1.5 cun from midline of spine between T 7 and T 8
	BL 18	1.5 cun from midline of spine between T 9 and T 10
	BL 19	1.5 cun from midline of spine between T 10 and T 11
	BL 20	1.5 cun from midline of spine between T 11 and T 12
	BL 21	1.5 cun from midline of spine between T 12 and L 1
	BL 22	1.5 cun from midline of spine between L 1 and L 2
	BL 23	1.5 cun from midline of spine between L 2 and L 3
	BL 24	1.5 cun from midline of spine between L 3 and L 4
	BL 25	1.5 cun from midline of spine between L 4 and L 5
	BL 26	1.5 cun from midline of spine between L 5 and S 1
	BL 27	1.5 cun from midline of spine at level of 1st sacral foramen
	BL 28	1.5 cun from midline of spine at level of 2nd sacral foramen
	BL 29	1.5 cun from midline of spine at level of 3rd sacral foramen

Meridian	Acupuncture Point	Location
Urinary Bladder Meridian (BL)	BL 30	1.5 cun from midline of spine at level of 4th sacral foramen
	BL 31	1 cun from midline of spine in 1st sacral foramen
	BL 32	1 cun from midline of spine in 2nd sacral foramen
	BL 33	1 cun from midline of spine in 3rd sacral foramen
	BL 34	1 cun from midline of spine in 4th sacral foramen
	BL 35	0.5 cun lateral to midline of spine on level with upper border of coccyx
	BL 41	3 cun from midline of spine between T 2 and T 3
	BL 42	3 cun from midline of spine between T 3 and T 4
	BL 43	3 cun from midline of spine between T 4 and T 5
	BL 44	3 cun from midline of spine between T 5 and T 6
	BL 45	3 cun from midline of spine between T 6 and T 7
	BL 46	3 cun from midline of spine between T 7 and T 8
	BL 47	3 cun from midline of spine between T 9 and T 10
	BL 48	3 cun from midline of spine between T 10 and T 11
	BL 49	3 cun from midline of spine between T 11 and T 12
	BL 50	3 cun from midline of spine between T 12 and L 1
	BL 51	3 cun from midline of spine between L 1 and L 2
	BL 52	3 cun from midline of spine between L 2 and L 3
	BL 53	3 cun from midline of spine at S 2 level
	BL 54	3 cun from midline of spine at S 4 level
Conception Meridian (CV)	CV 1	midpoint between anus and scrotum or posterior commissure of vulva
Gallbladder Meridian (GB)	GB 21	midpoint between GV 14 and lateral margin of acromion
Triple Heater Meridian (TH)	TH 15	1 cun inferior to GB 21 and 1 cun superior to SI 13

Meridian	Acupuncture Point	Location
Small Intestine Meridian (SI)	SI 9	1 cun superior to posterior axillary fold
	SI 10	3 cun superior to SI 9
	SI 11	midpoint between SI 12 and inferior angle of the scapula
	SI 12	midpoint of supraspinatus fossa
	SI 13	medial corner of supraspinatus fossa
	SI 14	3 cun from midline of spine between T 1 and T 2
	SI 15	2 cun from midline of spine between C 7 and T 1

Extra-Meridian Points

Table 14-2

Acupuncture Point	Location
Extra GV Point (interspinal)	add Extra GV point to midline of spine between T 2 and T 3, T 4 and T 5, T 8 and T 9 spinous processes
Extra Urinary Bladder point (paraspinal 1.5 cun)	add Extra BL point 1.5 cun between T 8 and T 9
	add Extra BL point 3 cun from midline of spine between T 8 and T 9
Huatuojiaji point (paraspinal 0.5 cun)	0.5 cun from midline of spine at all spinal segments (same as in neck)
Facet Joint point (paraspinal 1.0 cun)	1 cun from midline of spine at all spinal segments (same as in neck)
Yaoyi	3 cun from midline of spine at L 4 and L 5
Sacroiliac Joint point*	Upper Sacroiliac point: 2 cun from midline of spine at L 5 – S 1 (superior to posterior superior iliac spine)
	Lower Sacroiliac point: 2 cun from midline of spine at S 1 – S 2 (inferior to posterior superior iliac spine, Dimple of Venus)
Jian-Tung	midpoint of the lateral border of scapula

*Sacroiliac Joint

- between sacrum and two ilia
- small range of motion
- upper one-third bound by ligaments – sprain
- lower two-thirds synovial joint – arthritis (ankylosing spondylitis, rheumatoid arthritis, juvenile rheumatoid arthritis, psoriatic arthritis, or Reiter's disease)

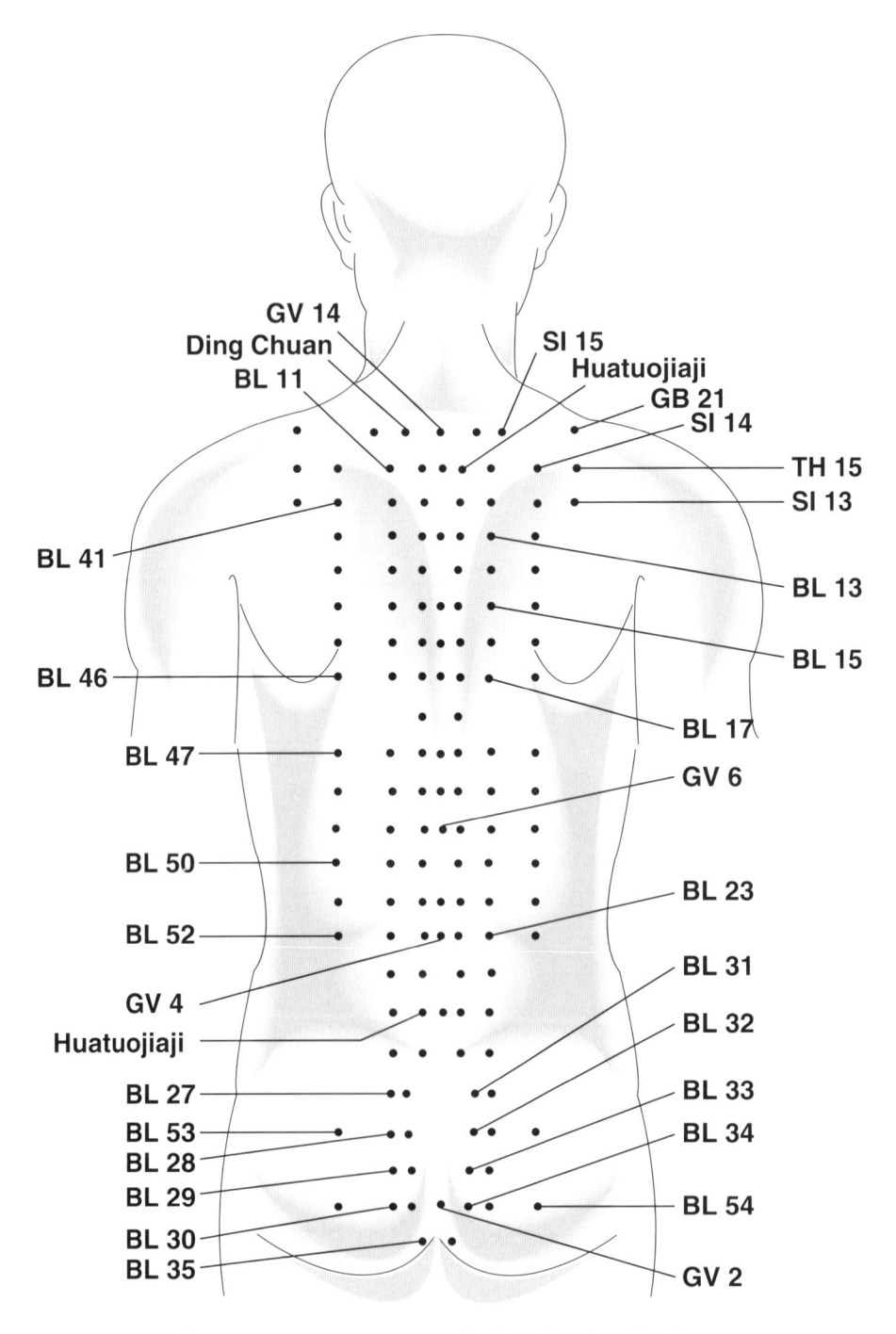

Fig. 14-1. Acupuncture Points in the Back - Surface View

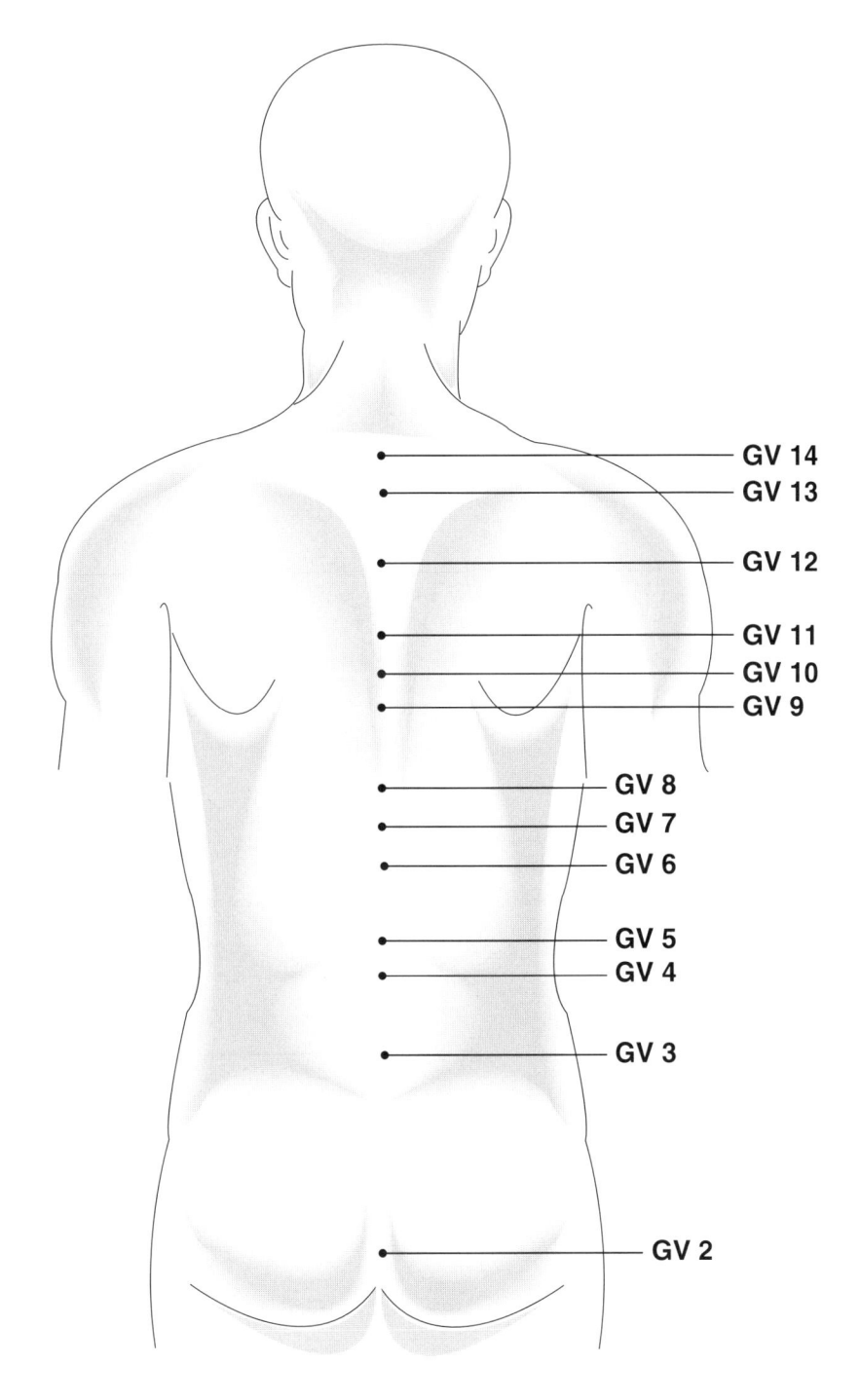

Fig. 14-2. Acupuncture Points in the Back
- GV Meridian Points

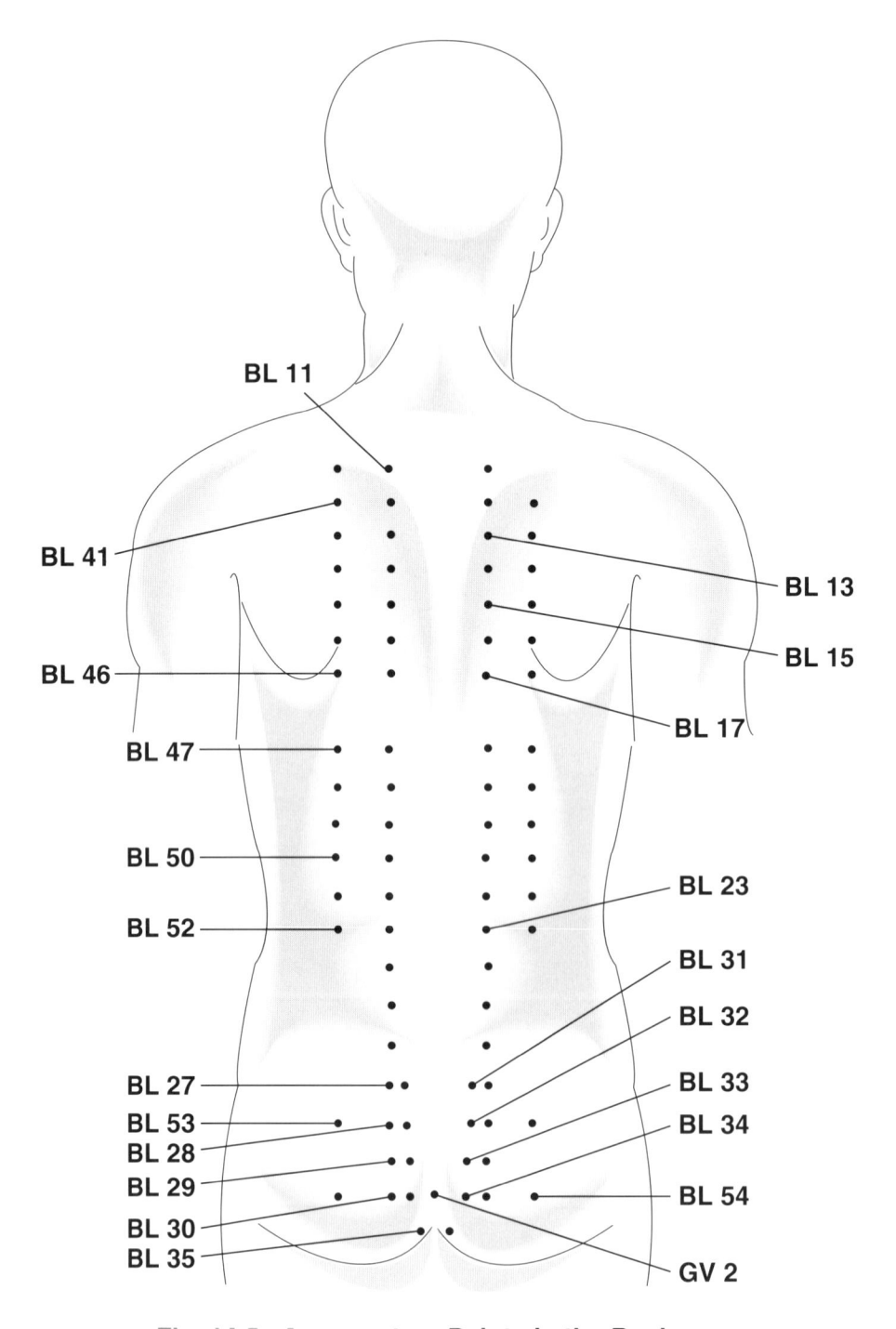

Fig. 14-3. Acupuncture Points in the Back
- BL Meridian Points

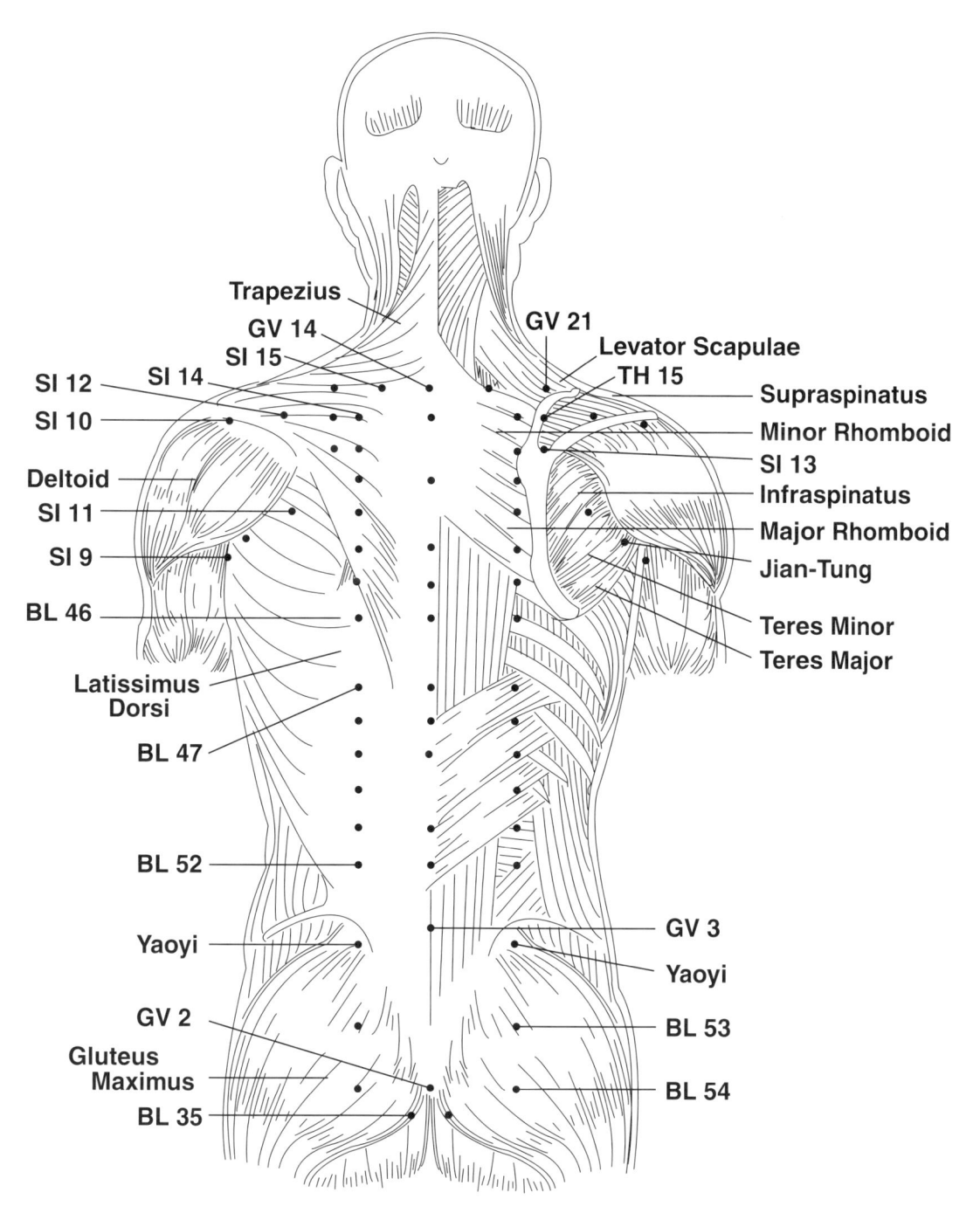

Fig. 14-4. Acupuncture Points in the Back - Superficial View

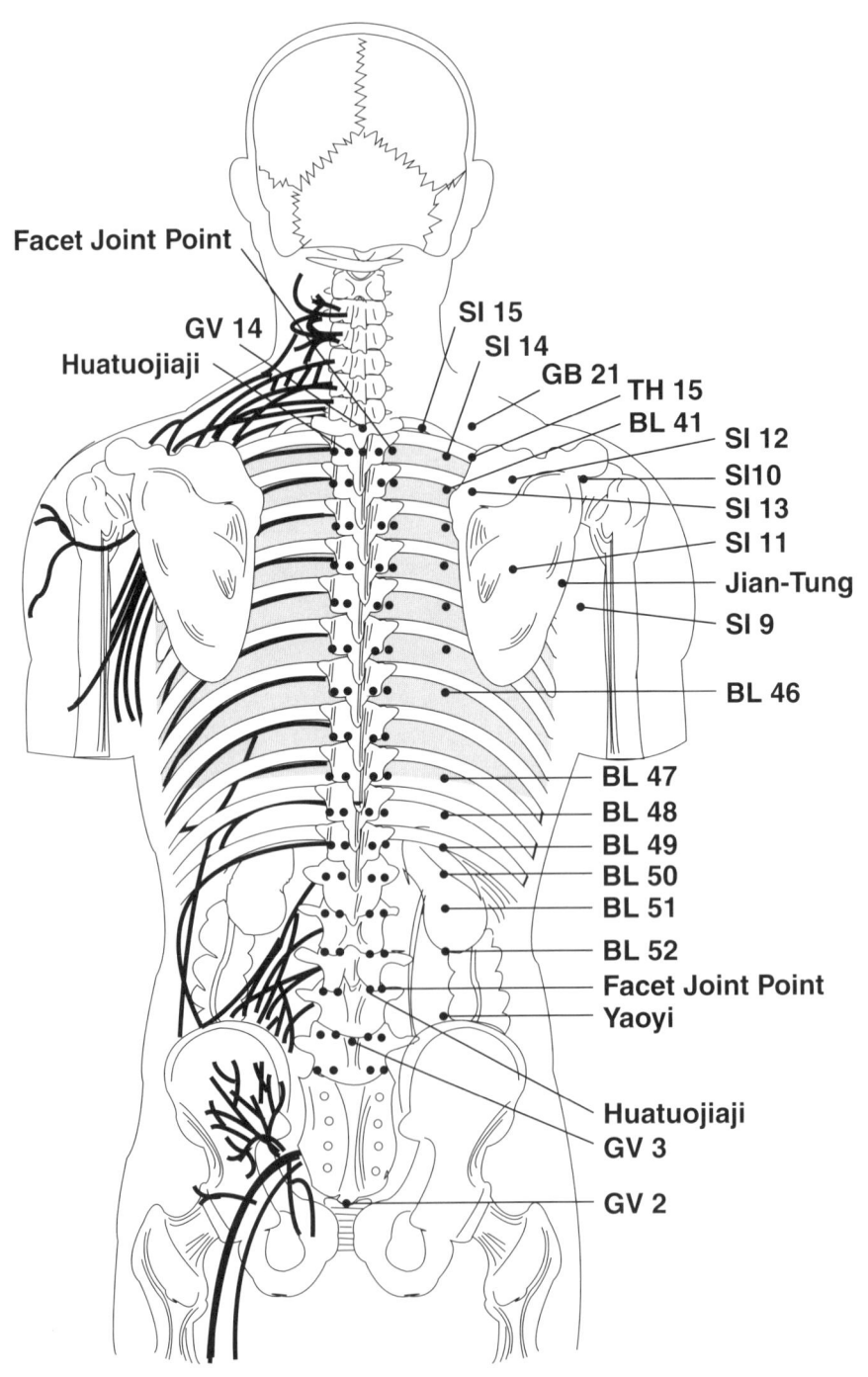

Fig. 14-5. Acupuncture Points in the Back
- Deep View

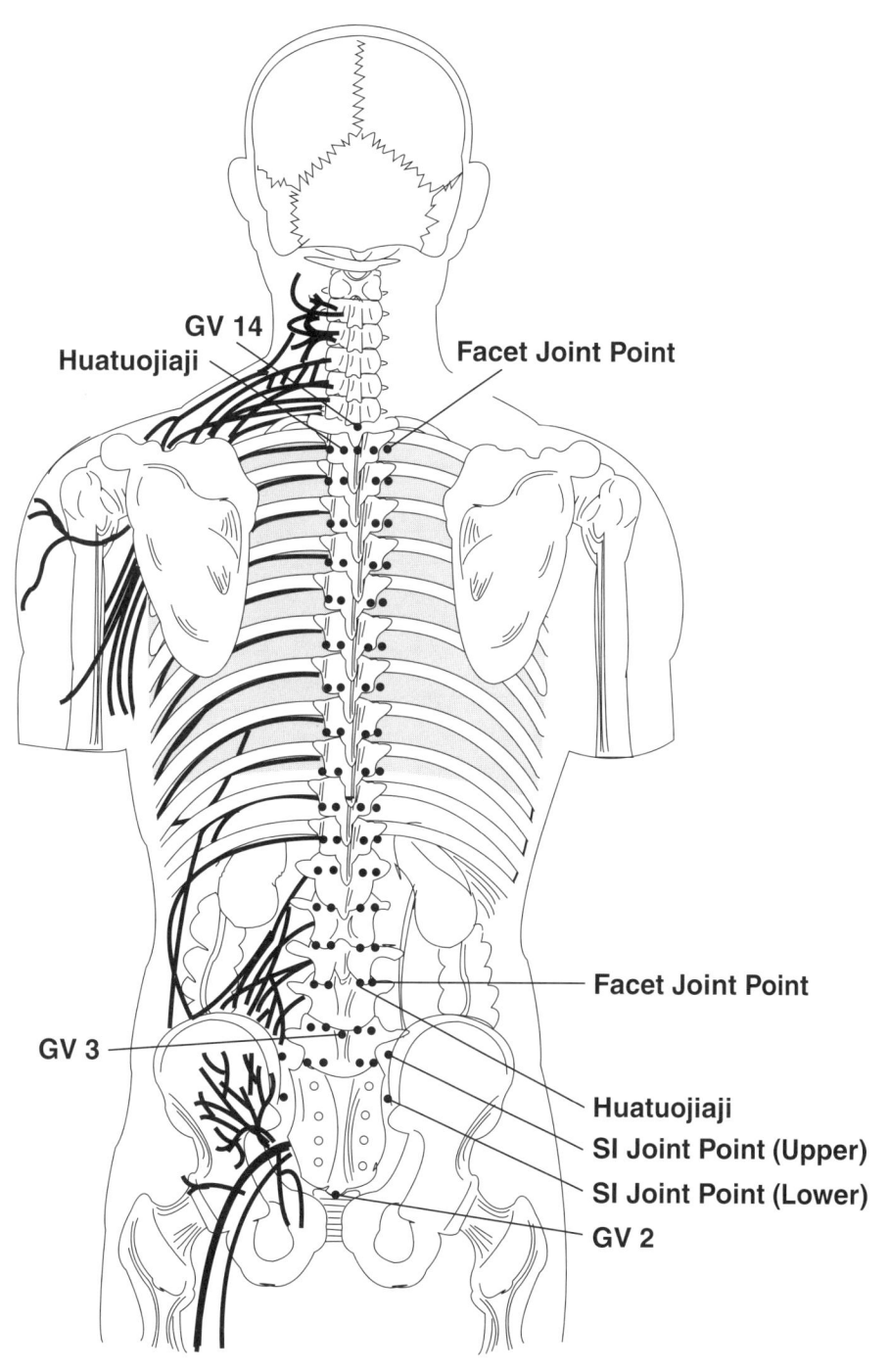

Fig. 14-6. Extra-Meridian Points in the Back
- Deep View

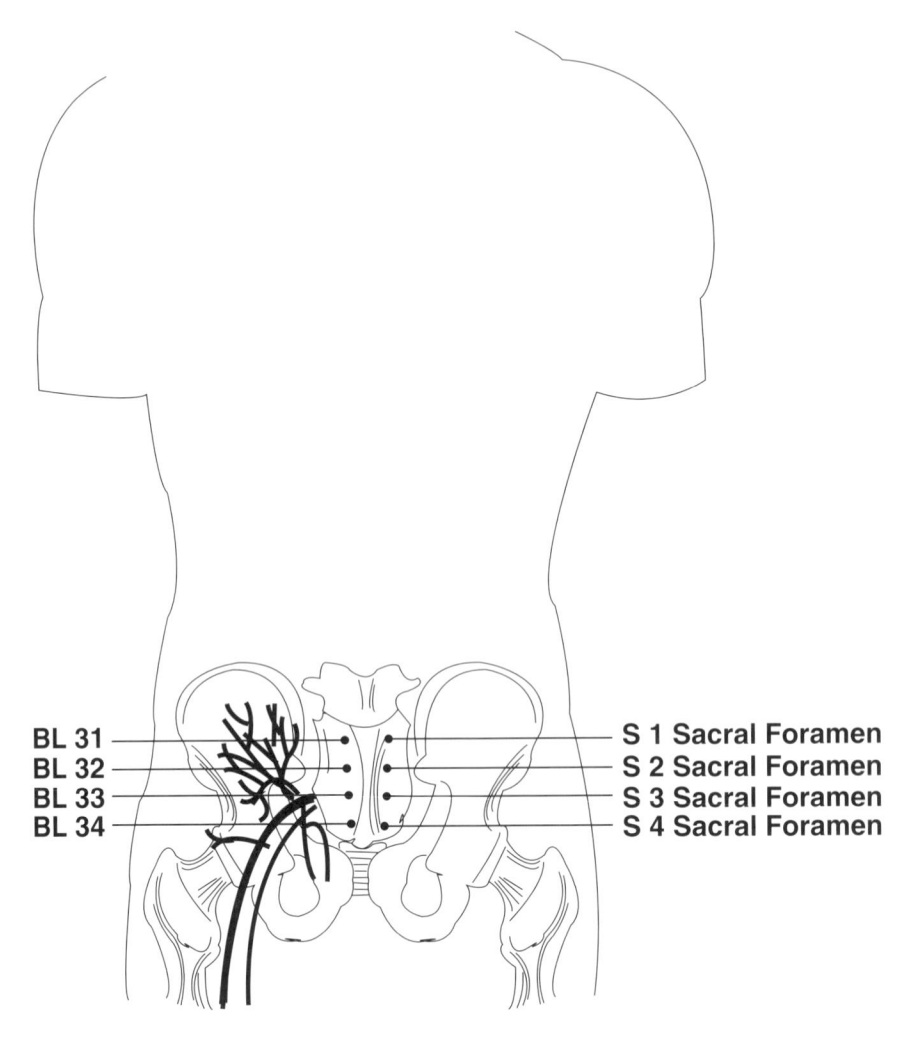

Fig. 14-7. Sacral BL Points in the Sacral Foramen

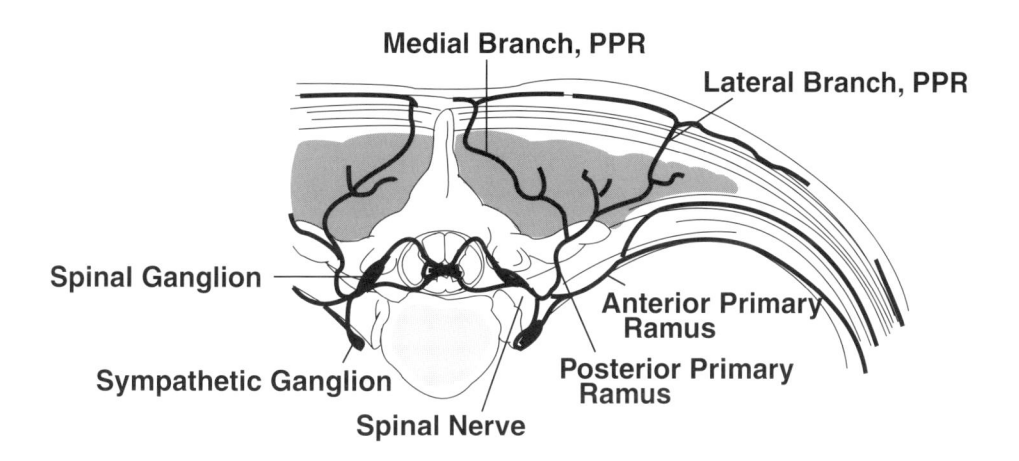

GV meridian point stimulates medial branch, posterior primary ramus.

BL meridian point (paraspinal 1.5 cun) stimulates lateral branch, posterior primary ramus.

BL meridian point (paraspinal 3.0 cun) stimulates anterior primary ramus.

Deep insertion of BL meridian point (paraspinal 1.5 cun) stimulates sympathetic ganglion.

Fig. 14-8. Nerve Stimulation of the Spine

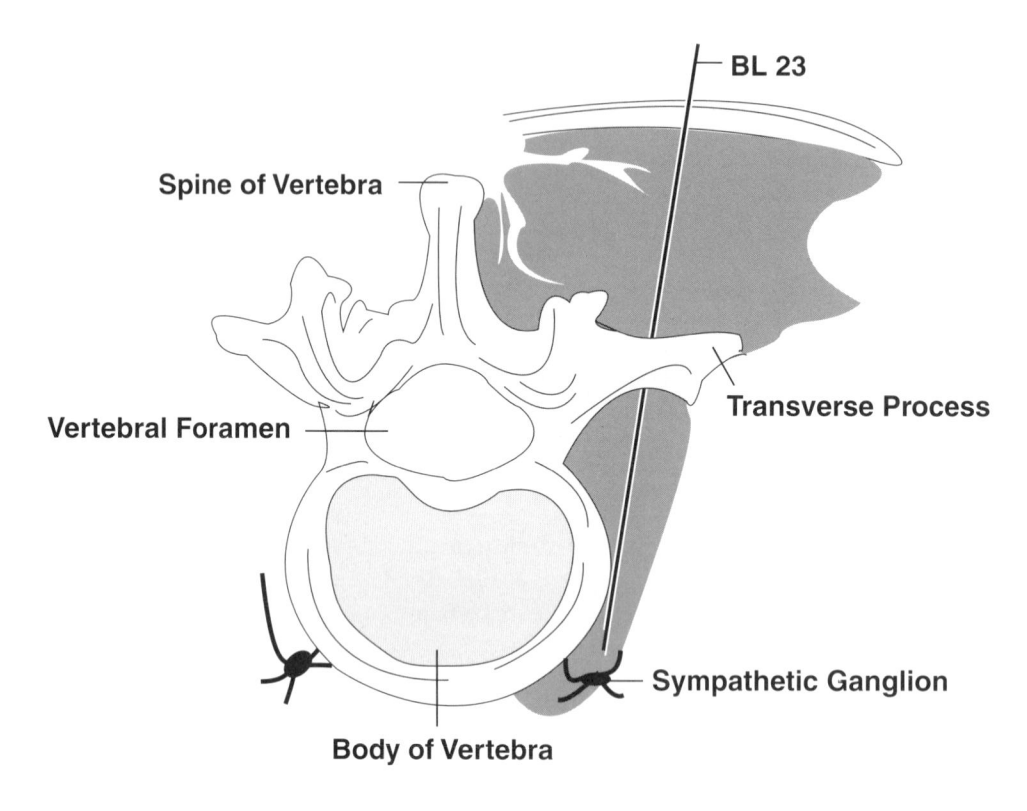

BL 23
Spine of Vertebra
Vertebral Foramen
Transverse Process
Sympathetic Ganglion
Body of Vertebra

Deep insertion of BL meridian point (paraspinal 1.5 cun) stimulates sympathetic ganglion.

Fig. 14-9. Stimulation of Sympathetic Ganglion

Nerve Stimulation in the Back

Table 14-3

	Name of Nerve	**Acupuncture Point**
Cranial Nerve	accessory nerve	GB 21
Spinal Nerve	medial branch of posterior primary ramus	GV 3 to GV 14
	lateral branch of primary ramus	BL 11 to BL 30
	anterior primary ramus	BL 41 to BL 52
	sinu-vertebral nerve	Huatuojiaji points at all spinal segments
	sacral spinal nerve	BL 27, BL 28, BL 29, BL 30, BL 31, BL 32, BL 33, BL 34
Peripheral Nerve	dorsal scapular nerve	SI 14, SI 15
	lower subscapular nerve	extra-meridian point Jian-Tung
	suprascapular nerve	SI 11, SI 12
	thoraco-dorsal nerve	BL 45 to BL 50
	superior clunial nerve	extra-meridian point, Yaoyi
	coccygeal nerve	BL 35
	superior gluteal nerve	BL 53
	inferior gluteal nerve	BL 54
	perineal nerve	GB 1, CV 1

Scapular Muscles

Table 14-4

Muscle	Action	Innervation Peripheral Nerve	Innervation Spinal Segment	Acupuncture Point
Rhomboid Minor	draws scapula upward and medially; depresses shoulder	dorsal scapular nerve	C 4, C 5	SI 14, SI 15
Rhomboid Major	draws scapula upward and medially; depresses shoulder	dorsal scapular nerve	C 5, C 6	SI 14, SI 15
Levator Scapulae	draws scapula upward	C 3, C 4 spinal nerves	C 3, C 4	SI 13, TH 15, GB 21, Spinal Nerve points C 3, C 4
Supraspinatus	abducts arm	suprascapular nerve	C 4 - C 6	SI 12, LI 16
Infraspinatus	rotates arm laterally	suprascapular nerve	C 4 - C 6	SI 11, LI 16
Teres Minor	rotates arm laterally	axillary nerve	C 4, C 5	TH 14, LI 15, SI 16
Teres Major	adducts, extends and rotates arm medially	lower scapular nerve	C 5 - C 8	Jian-Tung
Subscapularis	rotates arm medially	subscapular nerve	C 5 - C 7	Jubi
Serratus Anterior	pulls scapula forward	long thoracic nerve	C 5 - C 7	SP 21, GB 22

Acupuncture Point	Location
SP 21	mid-axillary line, 6 cun inferior to axillary fold
GB 22	mid-axillary line, 3 cun inferior to axillary fold

Trunk Muscles

Table 14-5

Muscle	Action	Peripheral Nerve	Spinal Segment	Acupuncture Point
External Intercostal	elevates ribs enlarges thorax	intercostal nerve		BL 41 - BL 49
Internal Intercostal	contracts thorax	intercostal nerve		BL 41 - BL 49
Diaphragm	expands thorax compresses abdomen	phrenic nerve	C 3 - C 5	ST 17, BL 17
Levatores Costarum	bends spine laterally extends and rotates spine	intercostal nerve		BL 41 - BL 49
Transversus Thoracis	depresses ribs	2nd to 6th intercostal nerves		BL 41 - BL 45
Serratus Posterior Superior	raises ribs	1st to 4th intercostal nerves		SI 14, BL 41 - BL 43
Serratus Posterior Inferior	draws ribs outward	9th to 11th intercostal nerves		BL 47, BL 48, BL 49

Back Muscles

Table 14-6

Muscle	Action	Peripheral Nerve	Spinal Segment	Acupuncture Point
Erector Spinae (Iliocostalis, Longissimus, Spinalis)	extend and bend head and vertebral column to side	C 1 to L 5 posterior primary ramus (lateral branch)		BL point (paraspinal 1.5 cun) at the respective spinal segment
Transversalis (Semispinalis, Multifidus, Rotatores)	extend and rotate spine	C 1 to L 5 posterior primary ramus (medial branch)		GV point at the respective spinal segment

Perineum Muscles

Table 14-7

Muscle	Action	Peripheral Nerve	Spinal Segment	Acupuncture Point
Levator Ani	flexes coccyx, raises anus	S 4 nerve		BL 34, BL 30
Coccygeus	flexes and abducts coccyx	S 3 and S4 nerves		BL 33, BL 29, BL 34, BL 30
External Anal Sphincter	keeps anus closed	inferior hemorrhoidal nerve		BL 34, BL 35
Transversus Perinei Profundus	draws back central tendon of perineum	perineal nerve		GV 1, CV 2
Transversus Perinei Superficialis	fixes central tendon of perineum	perineal nerve		GV 1, CV 1

Clinical Application

Rhomboid Strain

- myofascial strain in upper back commonly involves rhomboid minor and rhomboid major muscles
- SI 14, SI 15 for dorsal scapular nerves
- BL 43, BL 44, BL 45 for the muscles

Intercostal Muscle Strain

- intercostal muscle damage follows direct contusion
- rule-out rib fracture
- breathing and other movements aggravate pain
- BL meridian point (paraspinal 3 cun) for the respective spinal segment (for example: BL 41 for T 2 - T 3 level)

Scheuermann's Disease

- vertebral osteochondritis in age 12 to 18 males
- lower thoracic vertebrae often involved
- BL meridian point (paraspinal 1.5 cun) and Huatuojiaji points for the respective spinal segment

Degeneration (Osteoarthritis) of Thoracic Spine

- lipping of vertebral body
- wedging of mid-thoracic vertebrae
- interspinal approach: GV meridian point for the respective spinal segment
- paraspinal approach: BL meridian point (paraspinal 1.5 cun BL points) for the respective spinal segment

Rheumatoid Arthritis

- costovertebral, costotransverse and zygapophyseal joints commonly affected
- interspinal approach with GV meridian point for the respective spinal segment
- paraspinal approach with BL meridian point (paraspinal 1.5 cun) for the respective spinal segment
- add immune mechanism points: LI 4, ST 36, BL 23, SP 10, SP 6 (see page 106)

Ankylosing Spondylitis

- thoracic pain and stiffness best helped with Huatuojiaji point for the respective spinal segment
- BL 23 relieves generalized back pain involving upper and lower back
- LU 1, LU 2 promote respiratory function
- treat sacroiliac joints with Sacroiliac Joint points

Acupuncture Point	Location
LU 1	1 cun inferior to LU 2
LU 2	medial to coracoid process immediately inferior to clavicle

Discogenic Problem of Lumbar Spine

- disc protrusion or disc prolapse result in low back pain
- sciatic pain commonly associated with degenerative disc disease involving L 4, L 5, S 1 or S 2
- interspinal approach with GV meridian point for the respective spinal segment
- paraspinal approach with BL meridian points (1.5 cun) for the respective spinal segment
- BL 54 stimulates sacral plexus and inferior gluteal nerve
- GB 30 stimulates sciatic nerve
- BL 40, BL 60 relieve radicular pain in lower extremities
- GV 26 and lumbago points in hand for acupuncture mobilization, manipulation or exercises

Acupuncture Point	Location
GV 26	superior to midpoint of philtrum
Lumbago # 1	on dorsum of hand, midpoint between 2nd and 3rd metacarpal bones
Lumbago # 2	on dorsum of hand, midpoint between 4th and 5th metacarpal bones

Sacroiliac Sprain

- directly insert needle into Upper Sacroiliac Joint point
- BL 31, BL 32 stimulate sacral spinal nerves; S 1, S 2, which usually innervate sacroiliac joints
- instant favorable response always expected
- BL 54, which stimulates sacral plexus, also of help

Thoraco-Lumbar Fascia Strain (Superficial)

- frequent site of acute low back pain
- rather generalized involving the thoraco-lumbar fascia
- extra-meridian point Yaoyi stimulates superior clunial nerve
- BL 23 controls sympathetic hypersensitivity

Musculo-Tendinous Pain of Low Back (Deep)

- concurrent segmental scoliosis may exist
- superficially erector spinae muscles involved
- deep transversalis muscles produce midline pain
- erector spinae muscles: BL meridian point (paraspinal 1.5 cun) for the respective spinal segment
- transversalis muscles: GV meridian point (interspinal) for the respective spinal segment
- deep paraspinal muscles: Huatuojiaji point for the respective spinal segment

Piriformis Syndrome

- deep tenderness over greater sciatic foramen and piriformis muscle
- may have gynecological or gastro-intestinal dysfunction
- negative neurological findings
- instant relief with BL 31, BL 32
- SP 6 helps regulate gynecological or gastro-intestinal dysfunction

Coccydynia

- inflammation of coccyx
- muscle spasm of coccygeus and levator ani muscles
- BL 34, BL 30 stimulate 4th sacral spinal nerve
- GV 2 stimulates coccygeal nerve

Anal Pain

- muscle spasm of anal muscles (external anal sphincter)
- may have motor dysfunction
- BL 34, BL 35 relieve pain and regulate anal function

Perineal Pain

- perineal pain may involve perinei muscles
- rule-out perineal neuralgia
- GV 1, CV 1 relieve both muscular pain and neuralgia

Chapter Fifteen

The Shoulder

Acupuncture Meridians and Points in the Shoulder

There are six meridians crossing the shoulder:

Table 15-1

Meridian	Acupuncture Point	Location
Large Intestine Meridian (LI)	LI 14	3 cun distal to LI 15 at insertion of deltoid muscle
	LI 15	inferior to anterior tip of acromion with arm in ***abduction position***
	LI 16	in depression medial to acromion
Triple Heater Meridian (TH)	TH 13	3 cun distal to TH 14
	TH 14	inferior to posterior tip of acromion with arm in ***abduction position***
Small Intestine Meridian (SI)	SI 9	1 cun superior to posterior axillary fold
	SI 10	3 cun superior to SI 9, intra-articular to shoulder joint
	SI 11	midpoint between SI 12 and inferior angle of scapula
	SI 12	midpoint of supraspinatus fossa
Lung Meridian (LU)	LU 2	medial to coracoid process and inferior to clavicle
	LU 3	3 cun inferior to anterior axillary fold at lateral border of biceps brachii muscle
	LU 4	1 cun distal to LU 3

Meridian	Acupuncture Point	Location
Pericardium Meridian (PC)	PC 2	2 cun inferior to anterior axillary fold between two heads of biceps brachii muscle
Heart Meridian (HT)	HT 1	midpoint of axillary fossa

Extra-Meridian Points

Table 15-2

Acupuncture Point	Location
Taijian	lateral to coracoid process, inferior to clavicle intra-articular to shoulder joint
Jubi	2 cun inferior to Taijian
Jian-Tung	midpoint of lateral border of scapula
Jian-Qian	1 cun superior to anterior axillary fold
Biceps Tendon point (longhead)	midpoint between greater and lesser tubercles of humerus (bicipital groove)
Rotator Cuff Common Tendon points	LI 15 and TH 14 **with arm hanging down in an anatomical position**

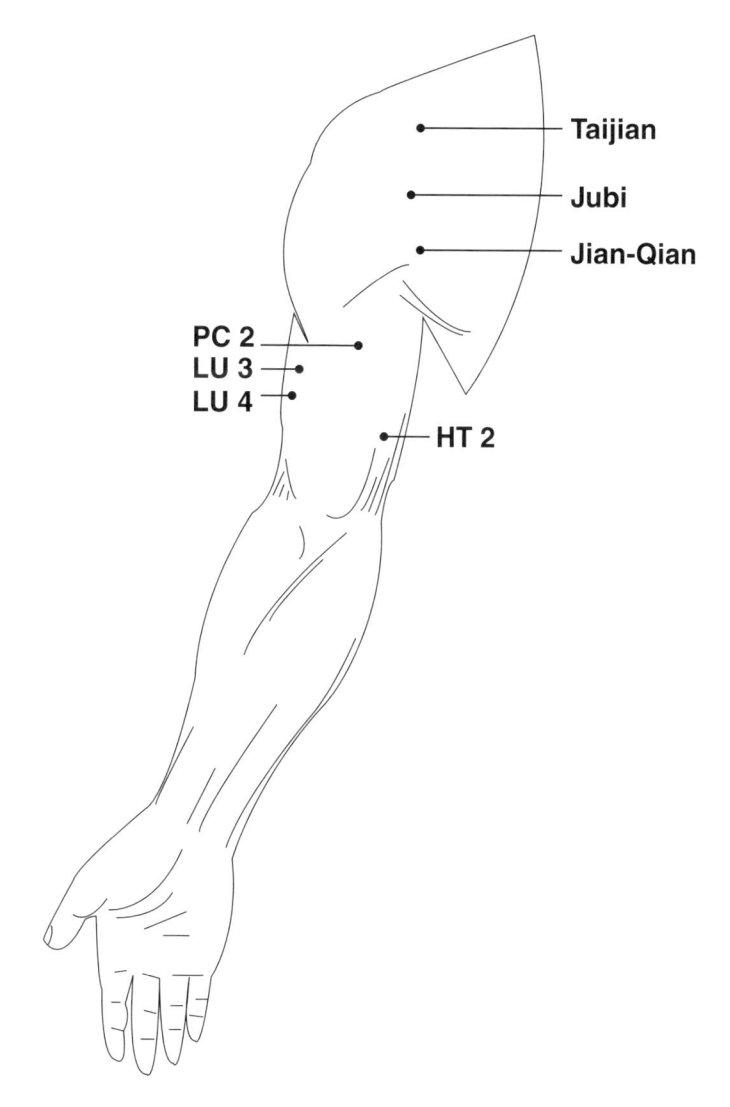

Fig. 15-1. Acupuncture Points in the Shoulder
 - Anterior Surface View

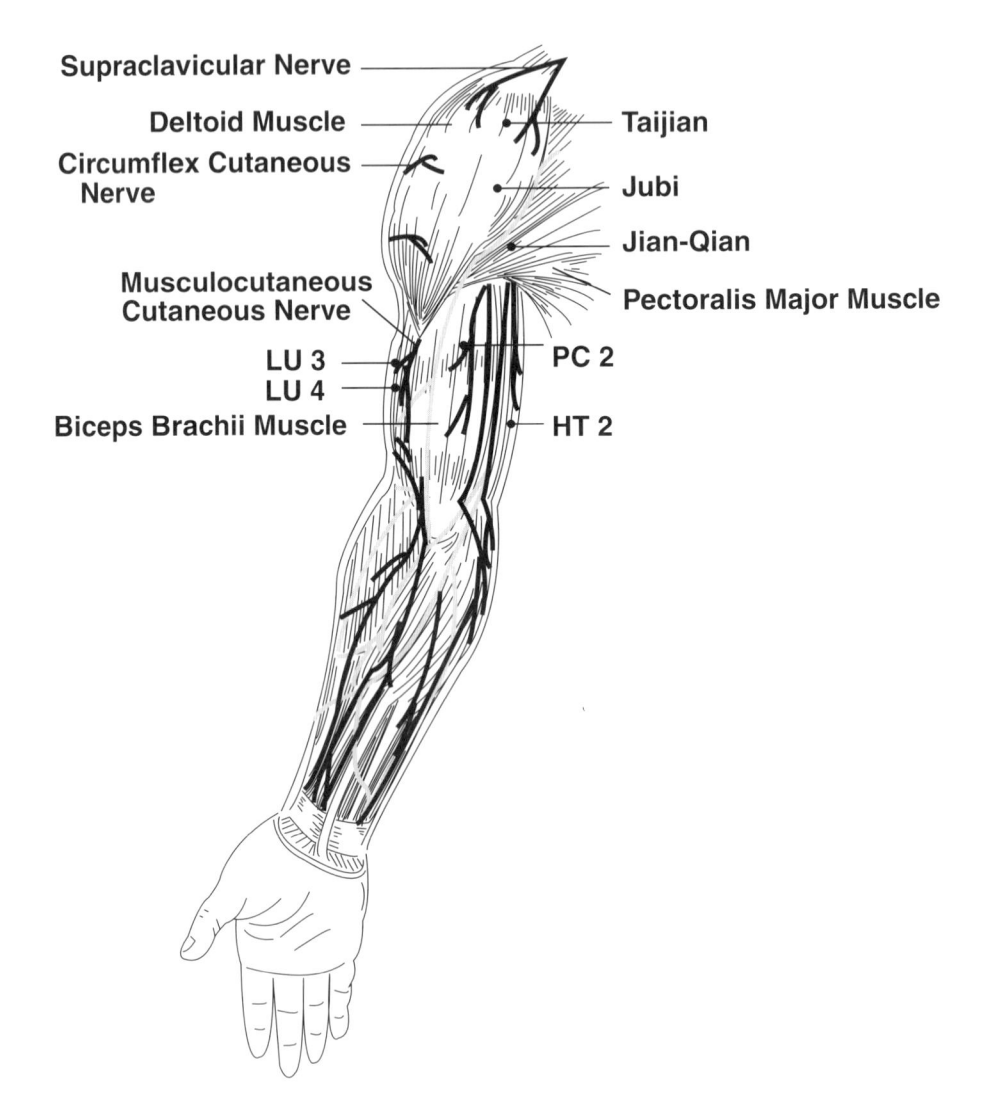

Fig. 15-2. Acupuncture Points in the Shoulder
  - Anterior Superficial View

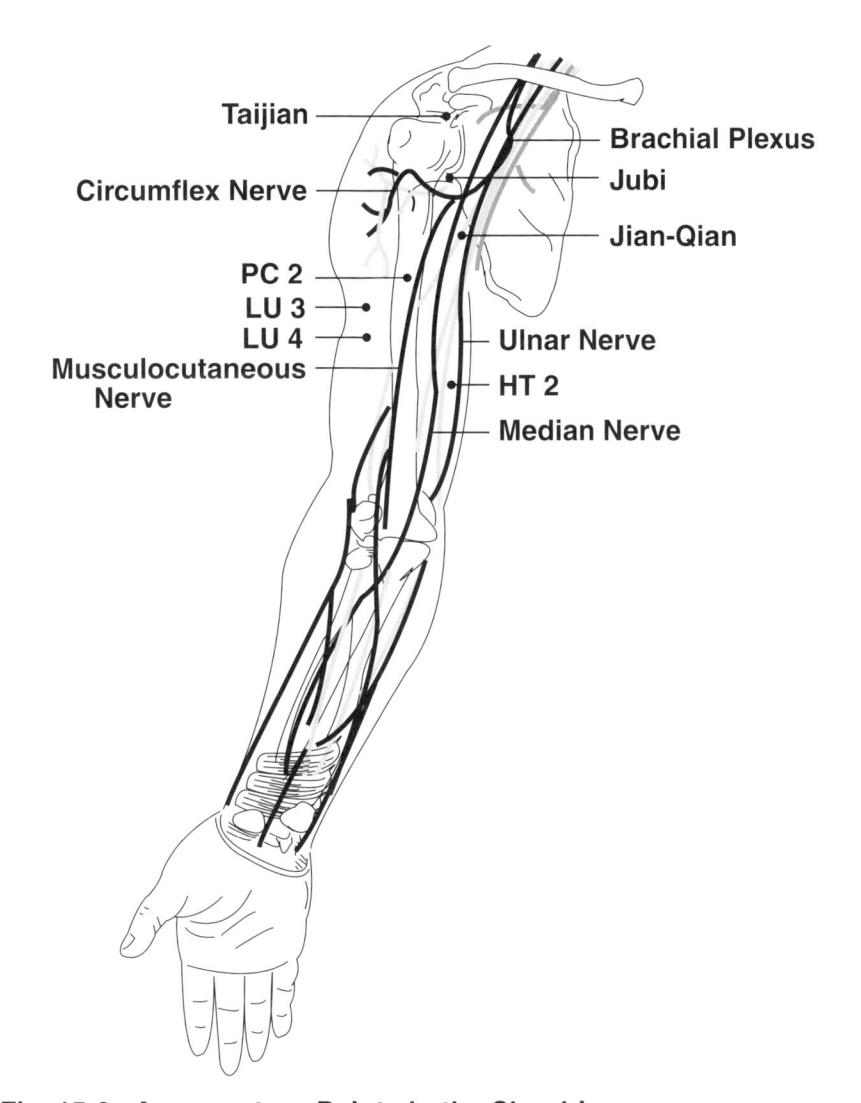

Fig. 15-3. Acupuncture Points in the Shoulder
 - Anterior Deep View

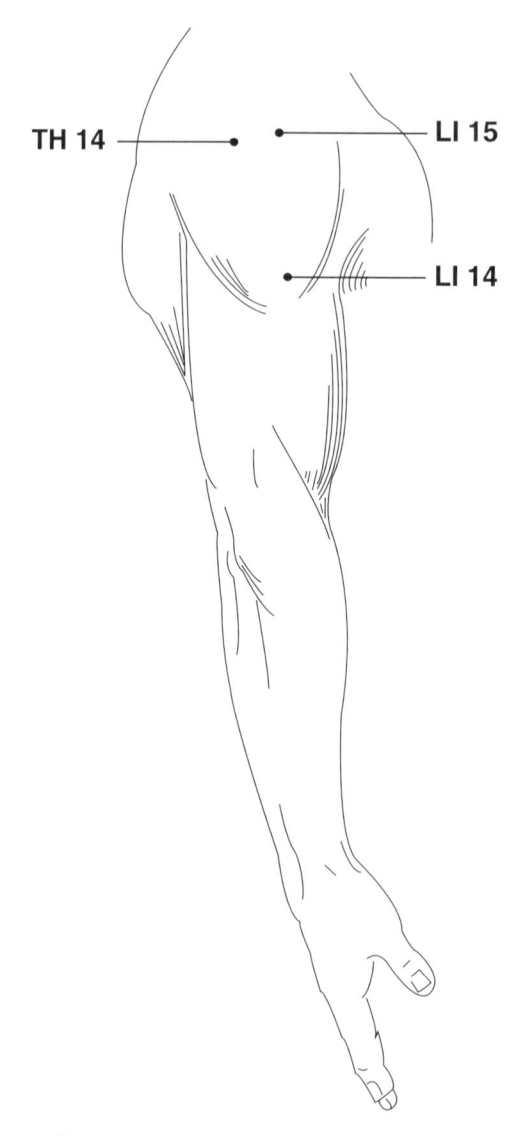

Fig. 15-4. Acupuncture Points in the Shoulder - Lateral Surface View

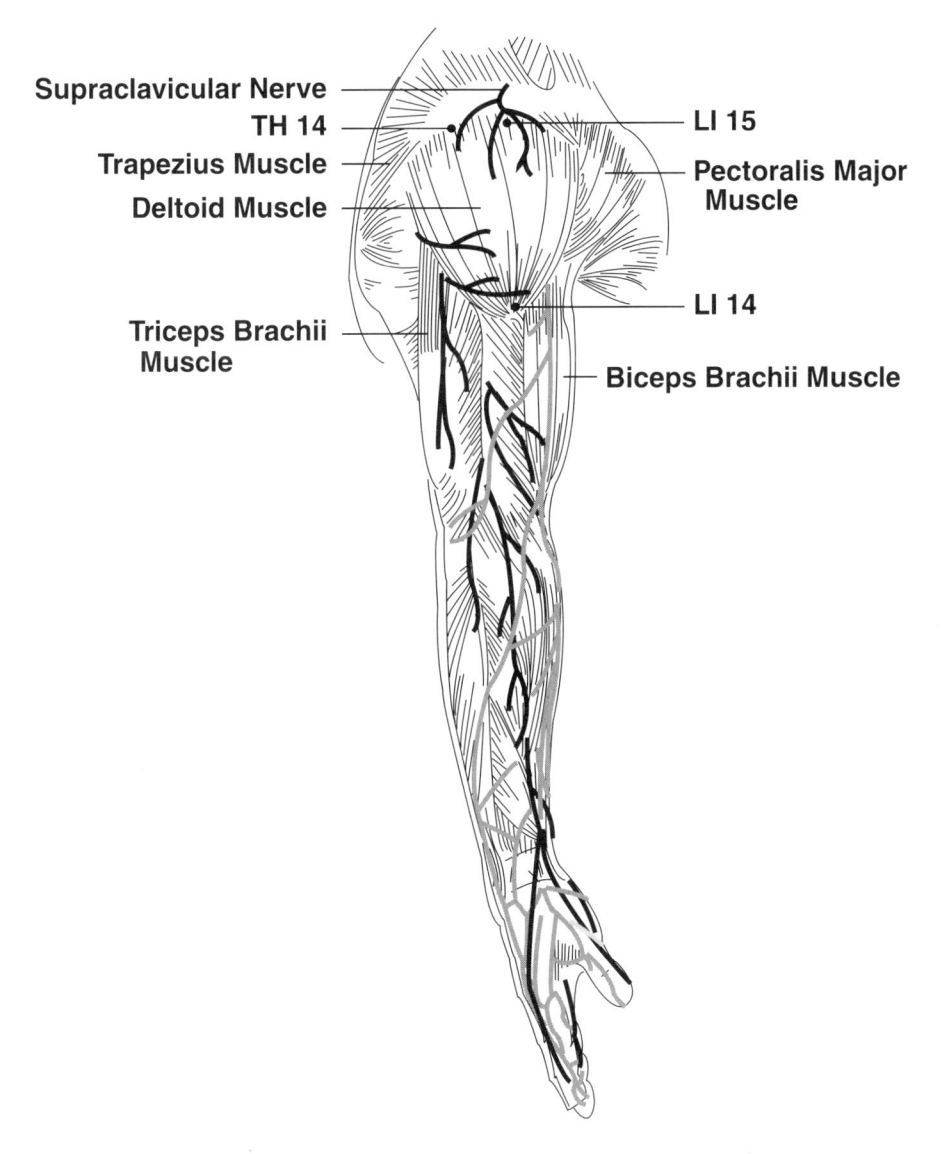

Fig. 15-5. Acupuncture Points in the Shoulder
- Lateral Superficial View

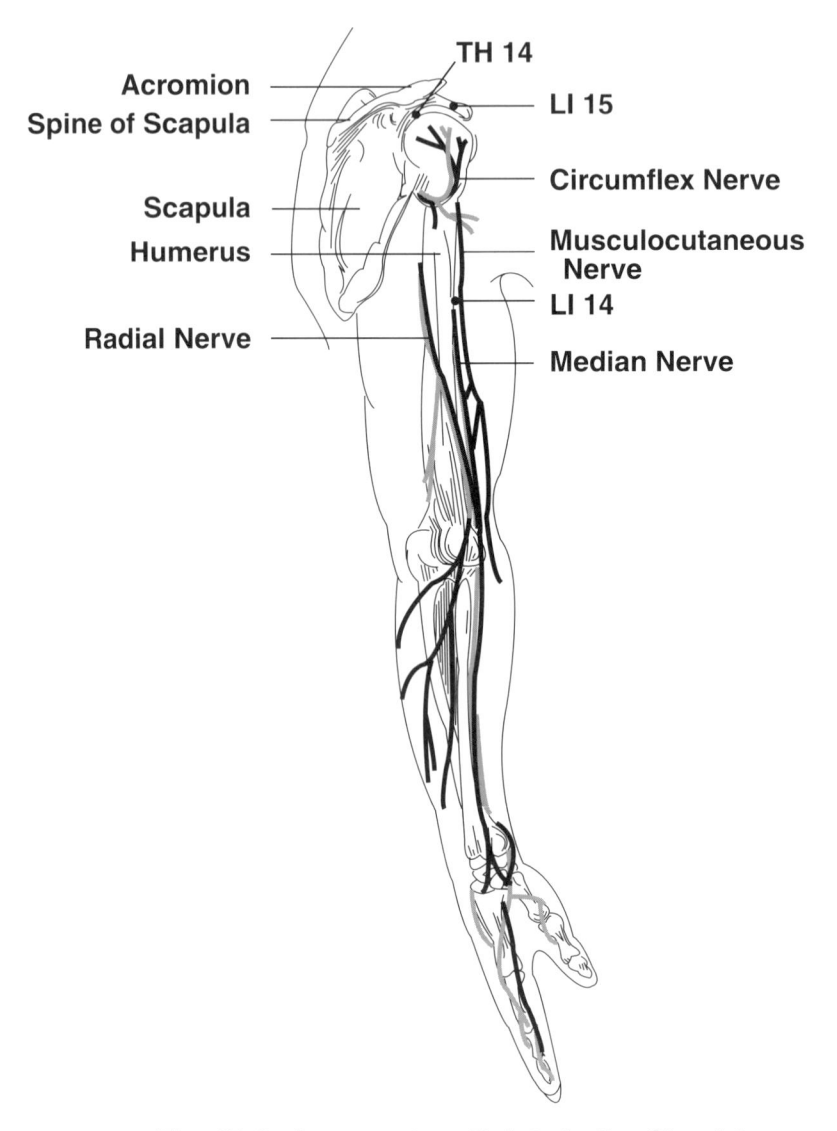

Fig. 15-6. Acupuncture Points in the Shoulder
- Lateral Deep View

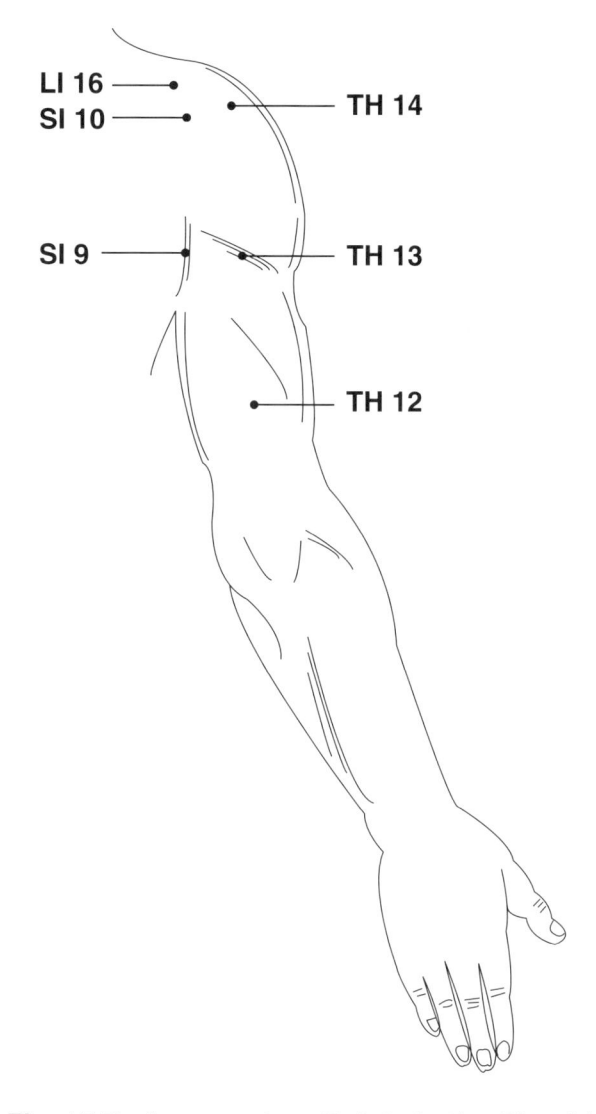

Fig. 15-7. Acupuncture Points in the Shoulder
- Posterior Surface View

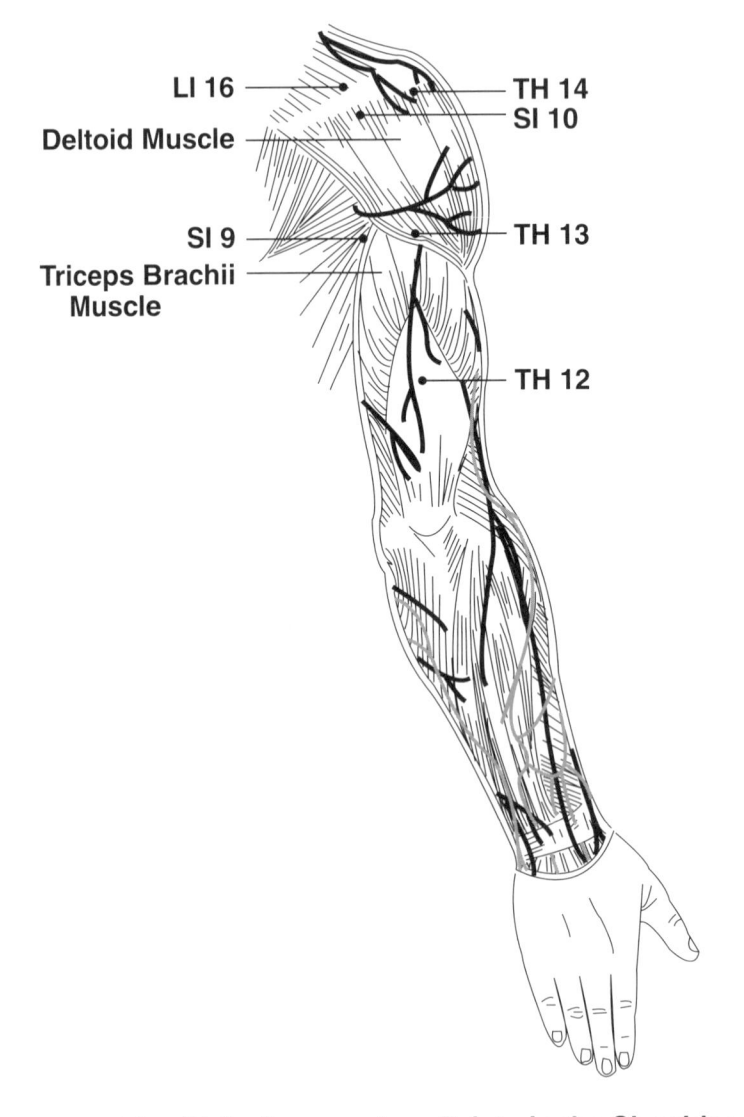

Fig. 15-8. Acupuncture Points in the Shoulder
- Posterior Superficial View

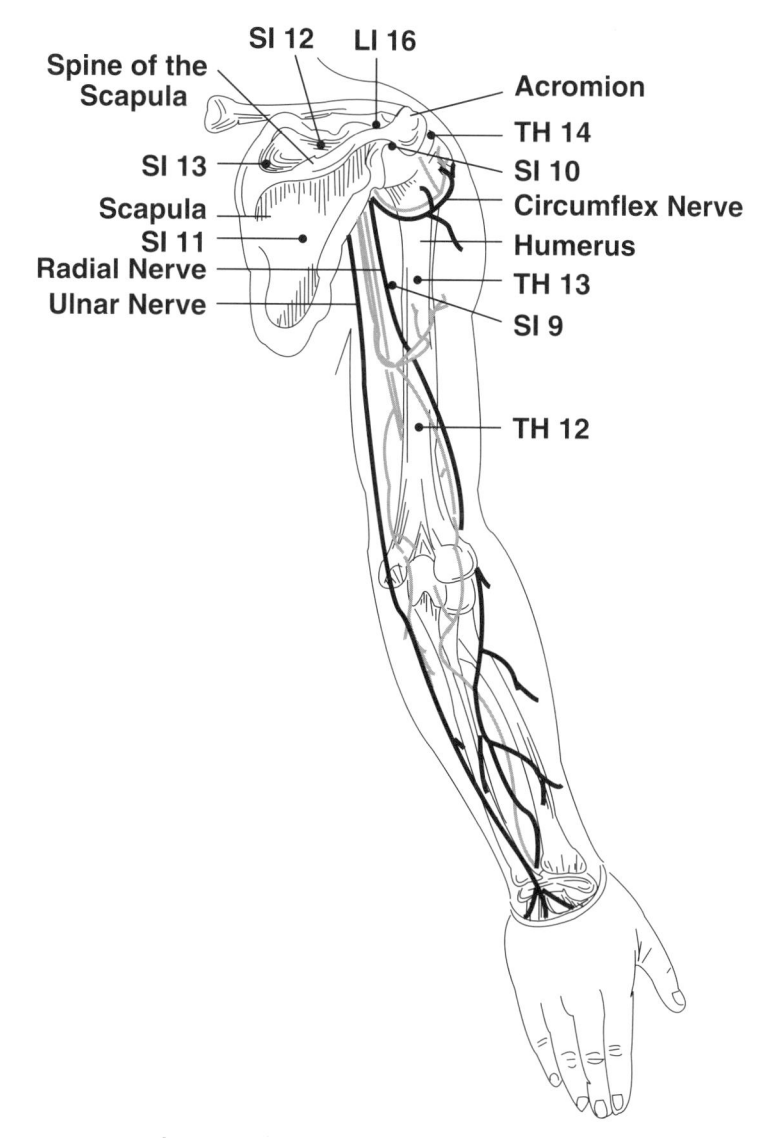

Fig. 15-9. Acupuncture Points in the Shoulder
- Posterior Deep View

Nerve Stimulation in the Shoulder

Table 15-3

	Name of Nerve	**Acupuncture Point**
Direct Stimulation to Shoulder	rotator cuff common tendon	LI 15, TH 14 **with arm hanging down in an anatomical position**
	shoulder joint (intra-articular)	Taijian (anterior), SI 10 (posterior)
	biceps tendon (long head)	midpoint between greater and lesser tubercles of humerus (bicipital groove)
Peripheral Nerve	axillary nerve	LI 15, TH 14, SI 9
	suprascapular nerve	SI 11, SI 12, SI 13, LI 16
	supraclavicular nerve	LI 16
	subscapular nerve	Jubi
	musculocutaneous nerve	LU 3, LU 4, PC 2
	anterior thoracic nerve	LU 2
	lower subscapular nerve	Jian-Tung
Neuro-Plexus	brachial plexus	HT 1, LU 2, Jian-Qian

Scapular Muscles *(see page 126)* and Shoulder Muscles

Table 15-4

Muscle	Action	Peripheral Nerve	Spinal Segment	Acupuncture Point
Coracobrachialis	adducts and flexes arm; rotates arm medially	musculocutaneous nerve	C 6, C 7	PC 2, LU 3, LU 4
Deltoid	adducts arm, anterior part flexes and rotates arm medially; posterior part extends and rotates arm laterally	axillary nerve	C 5, C 6	TH 14, LI 15, SI 10
Pectoralis Major	adducts, flexes and rotates arm medially	anterior thoracic nerve	C 5 - C 8, T 1	LU 2
Latissimus Dorsi	adducts, extends and rotates arm medially	thoracodorsal nerve	C 6 - C 8	GB 22, BL 46 - BL 52
Pectoralis Minor	pulls scapula forward	anterior thoracic nerve	C 6 - C 8	LU 1, LU 2
Biceps Brachii	flexes and rotates arm medially; long head abducts arm; short head adducts arm	musculocutaneous nerve	C 5, C 6	PC 2, LU 3, LU 4, bicipital groove point
Triceps Brachii	extends and adducts arm	radial nerve	C 7, C 8, T 1	SI 9, TH 13

(Innervation)

Clinical Application

Arthritis of the Shoulder

- shoulder joint may be affected by osteoarthritis or rheumatoid arthritis

- shoulder joint treated with intra-articular point, SI 10, and extra-meridian point, Taijian

- shoulder joint innervated by axillary nerve and treated with TH 14, LI 15, SI 10

- for rheumatoid arthritis add immune mechanism points: LI 4, ST 36, BL 23, SP 10, SP 6 (see page 106)

Acute Sub-Deltoid Bursitis

- acute shoulder pain with sudden onset

- bursa is extra-articular

- painful adduction of arm

- acupuncture points LI 14, LI 15, TH 14

Acromio-Clavicular Separation

- ligamentous strain or partial tear in type one

- minor subluxation if no instability in type two

- acupuncture points for type one and type two: LI 16, LU 2, extra-meridian point Taijian

- acromio-clavicular dislocation in type three usually requires surgery

Rotator Cuff Syndrome

- direct stimulation of rotator cuff common tendon: LI 15, TH 14, **with arm hanging downward in an anatomical position**

- peripheral nerve stimulation of axillary nerve: LI 15, TH 14, with arm in an **abducted and flexed position**

- peripheral nerve stimulation for individual muscles: SI 12 for supraspinatus, SI 11 for infraspinatus, SI 10 for teres minor

- deep insertion LI 16 affecting all these three muscles

Subscapularis Tendinitis

- this muscle originates in subscapular surface (invisible)
- tendon insertion at lesser tubercle of humerus (visible)
- extra-meridian point Jubi stimulates tendon insertion
- usually obvious improvement in medial rotation of arm

Bicipital Tendinitis

- pain and tenderness over bicipital groove
- painful arc usually present on shoulder forward flexion
- musculocutaneous nerve treated with PC 2, LU 3, LU 4
- also direct stimulation to Biceps Tendon point (extra-meridian)

Frozen Shoulder

- inflammatory changes and adhesion formation to shoulder
- fibrosis and retraction of capsule
- thickening of coraco-humeral ligament and subscapularis tendon
- primary frozen shoulder is idiopathic
- secondary frozen shoulder may be precipitated by trauma
- concurrent frozen shoulder may be associated with CVA, thyroid disease, cardiac disease, pulmonary disease, diabetes mellitus, hormonal dysfunction, thoracic surgery or emotional disorders

Stage 1 of Frozen Shoulder

- severe generalized pain and inflammation
- bursitis, tendinitis, periarthritis and capsulitis with sympathetic dysfunction
- acupuncture points: TH 5, LI 11, GB 34, ST 38
- control of upper extremity sympathetic dysfunction in the neck: ST 11
- spinal nerve pain control: Spinal Nerve point C 5

Stage 2 of Frozen Shoulder

- increase of shoulder movement limitations – adhesive capsulitis
- peripheral nerve stimulation for individual muscles according to limitation of movement (see Table 14-4 and Table 15-4)
- GV 26, GB 34 for acupuncture mobilization, manipulation or exercises

Stage 3 of Frozen Shoulder

- chronic adhesive capsulitis with retraction of capsule, thickening of ligaments and tendons and narrowing of joint space

- HT 1, LU 2, Jian-Qian for brachial plexus stimulation

- continue peripheral nerve stimulation for individual shoulder muscles

- continue acupuncture mobilization, manipulation or exercises

Chapter Sixteen

The Elbow and the Forearm

Acupuncture Meridians and Points in the Elbow and the Forearm

There are six meridians crossing the elbow and the forearm:

Table 16-1

Meridian	Acupuncture Point	Location
Large Intestine Meridian (LI)	LI 11	at lateral end of elbow crease, midpoint between lateral epicondyle and biceps aponeurosis in cubital fossa
	LI 10	2 cun distal to LI 11
	LI 12	1 cun proximal to LI 11
Triple Heater Meridian (TH)	TH 10	1 cun proximal to olecranon
	TH 9	5 cun distal to olecranon between ulna and radius
	TH 8	4 cun proximal to dorsal wrist crease
	TH 7	3 cun proximal to dorsal wrist crease on ulnar side of TH 6
	TH 6	3 cun proximal to dorsal wrist crease between ulna and radius
	TH 5	2 cun proximal to dorsal wrist crease between ulna and radius

Meridian	Acupuncture Point	Location
Small Intestine Meridian (SI)	SI 8	in elbow between olecranon and medial epicondyle
	SI 7	5 cun proximal to dorsal wrist crease
	SI 6	on radial side of styloid process of ulna
Lung Meridian (LU)	LU 5	on cubital crease on radial side of aponeurosis biceps brachii
	LU 6	5 cun distal to LU 5
Pericardium Meridian (PC)	PC 3	on cubital crease on ulnar side of aponeurosis biceps brachii
	PC 4	5 cun proximal to volar wrist crease
	PC 5	3 cun proximal to volar wrist crease
	PC 6	2 cun proximal to volar wrist crease between tendons of palmary longus and flexor carpi radialis
Heart Meridian (HT)	HT 3	on cubital crease midpoint between bicipital aponeurosis and medial epicondyle
	HT 4	1.5 cun proximal to palmar wrist crease on radial side of flexor carpi ulnaris muscle

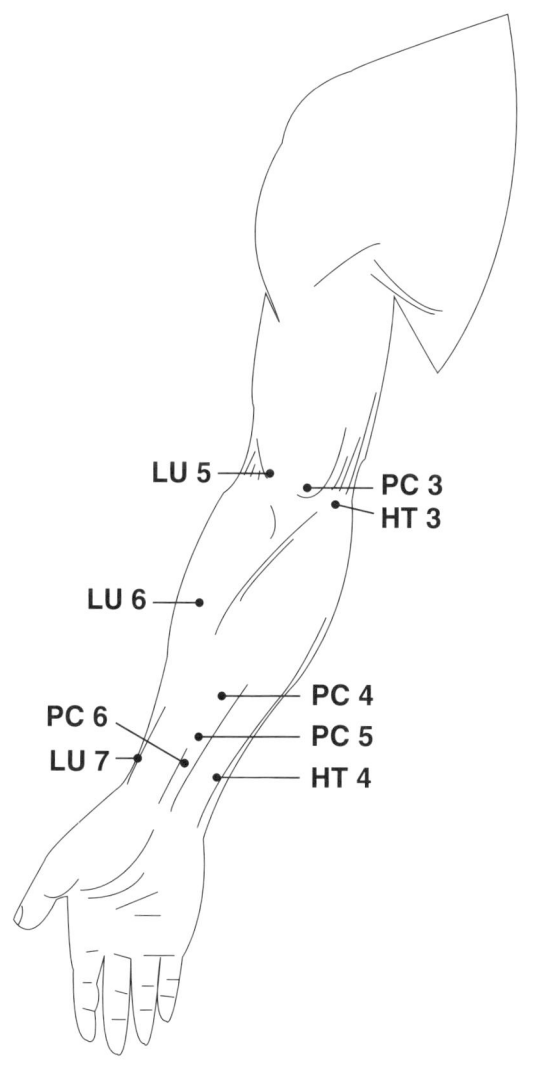

**Fig. 16-1. Acupuncture Points in the Elbow and the Forearm
 - Anterior Surface View**

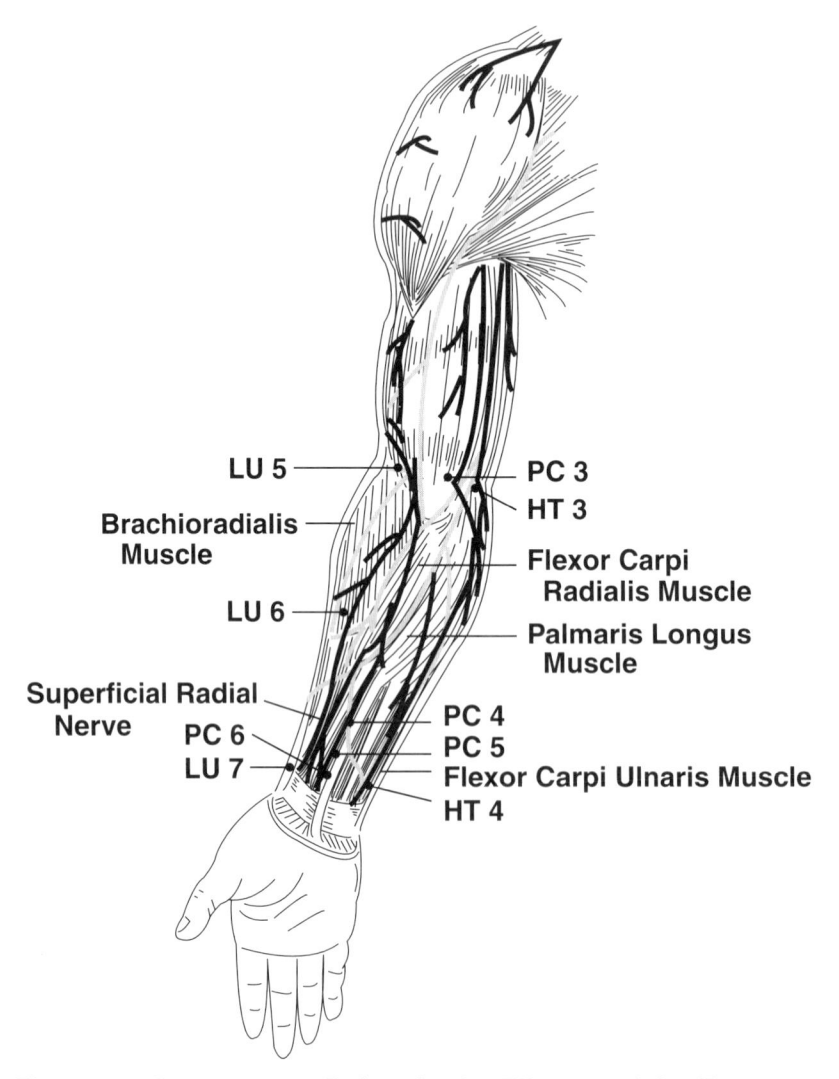

Fig. 16-2. Acupuncture Points in the Elbow and the Forearm
- Anterior Superficial View

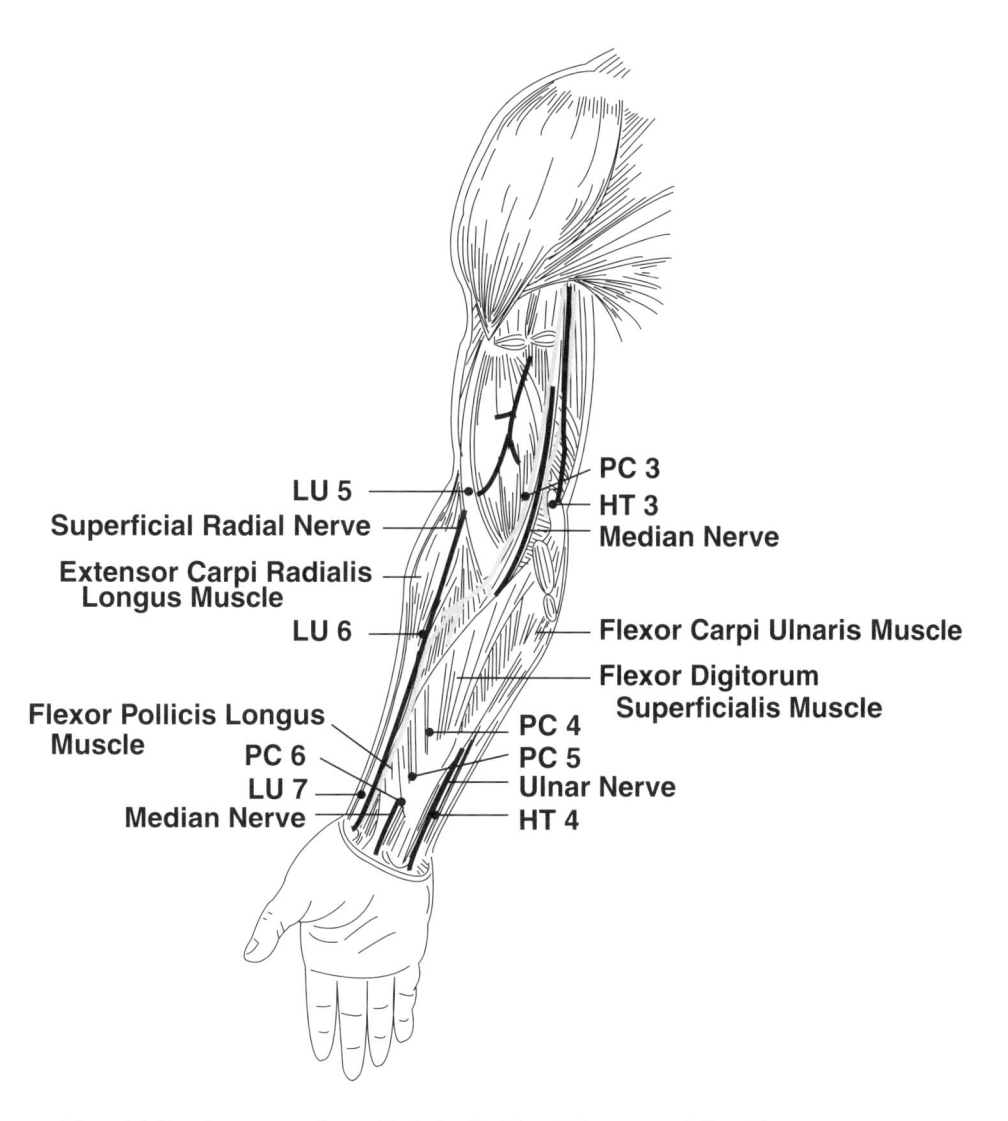

Fig. 16-3. Acupuncture Points in the Elbow and the Forearm
 - Anterior Middle View

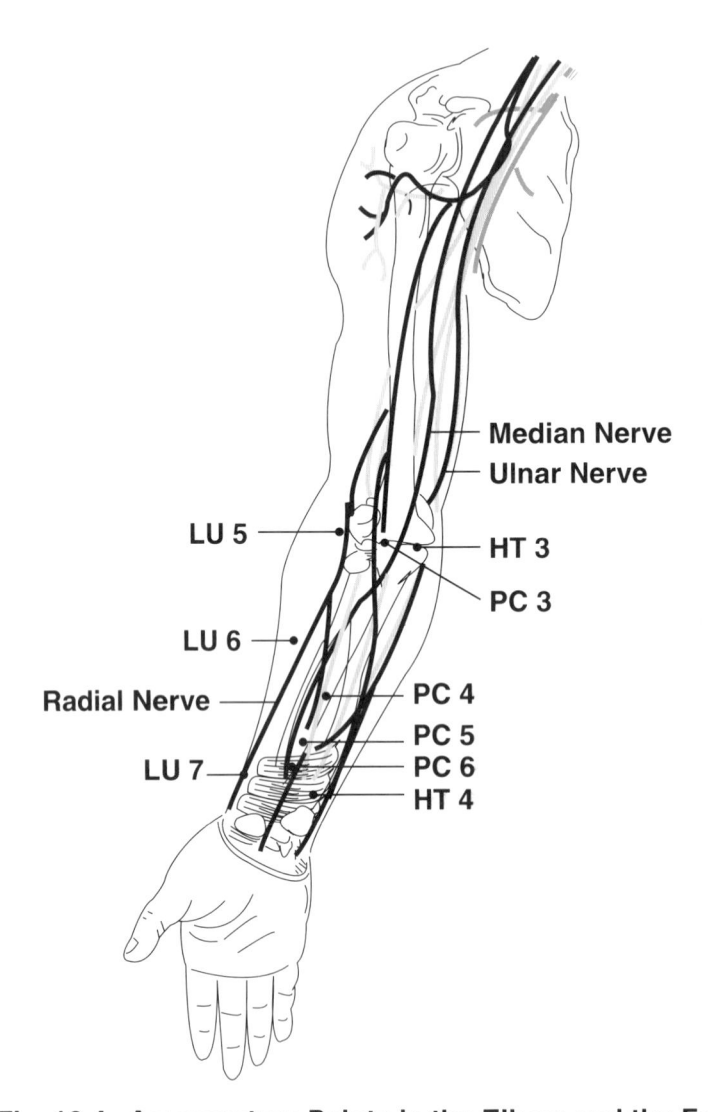

Fig. 16-4. Acupuncture Points in the Elbow and the Forearm
- Anterior Deep View

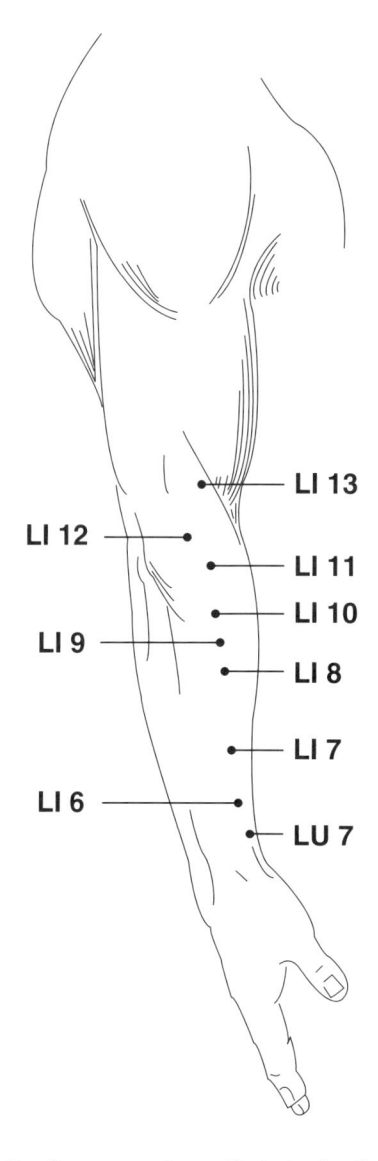

Fig. 16-5. Acupuncture Points in the Elbow and the Forearm
- Lateral Surface View

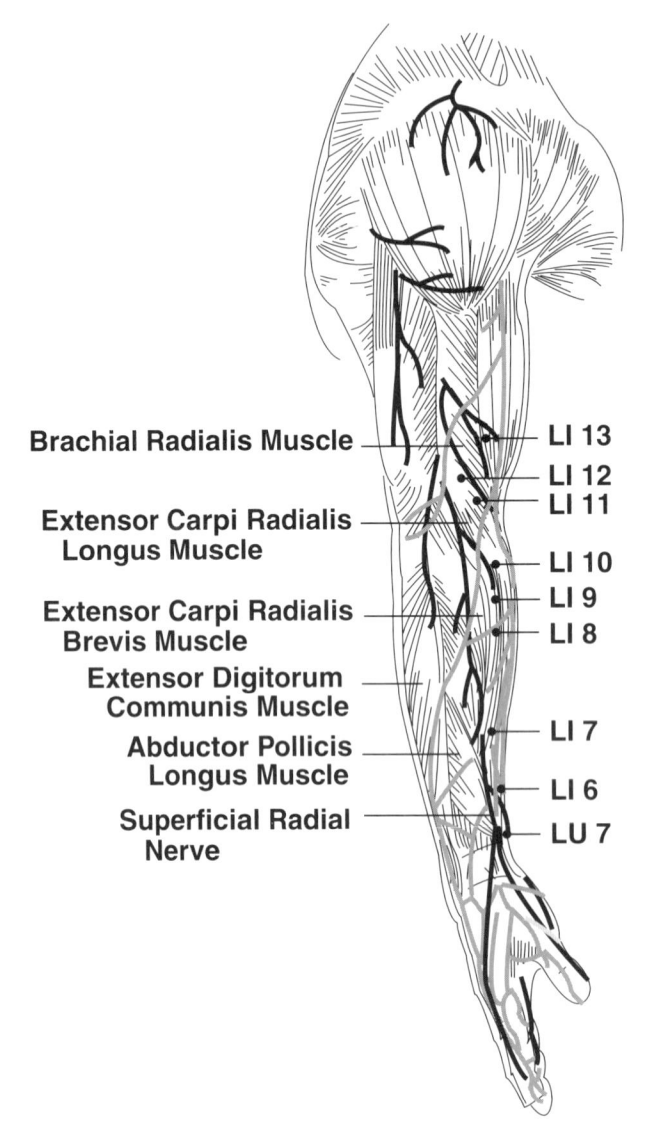

Fig. 16-6. Acupuncture Points in the Elbow and the Forearm
- Lateral Superficial View

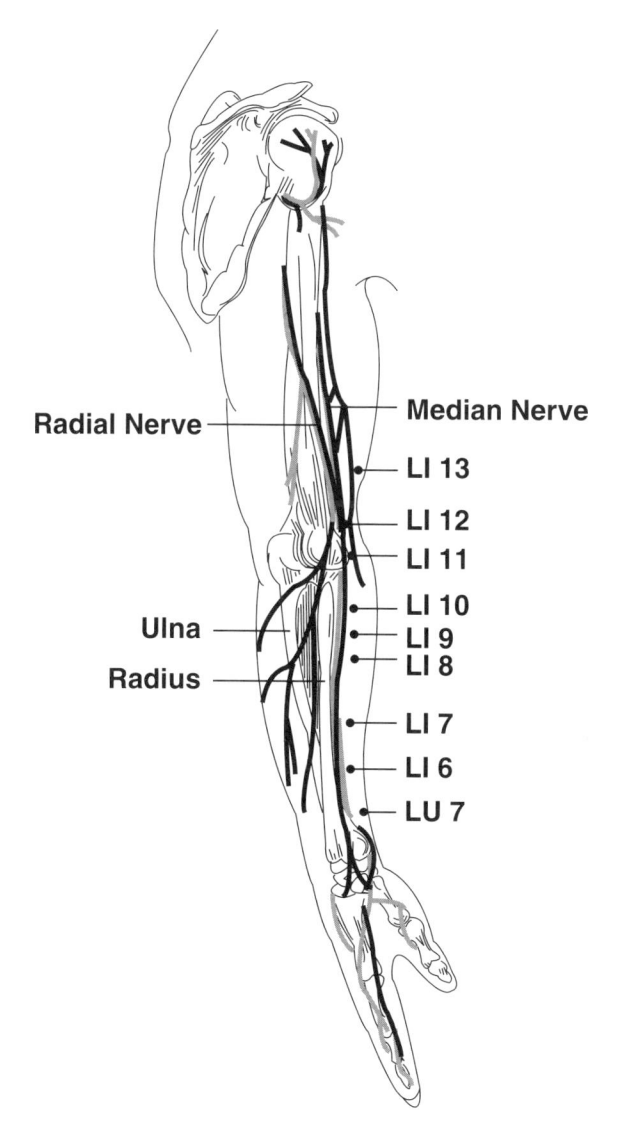

Fig. 16-7. Acupuncture Points in the Elbow and the Forearm - Lateral Deep View

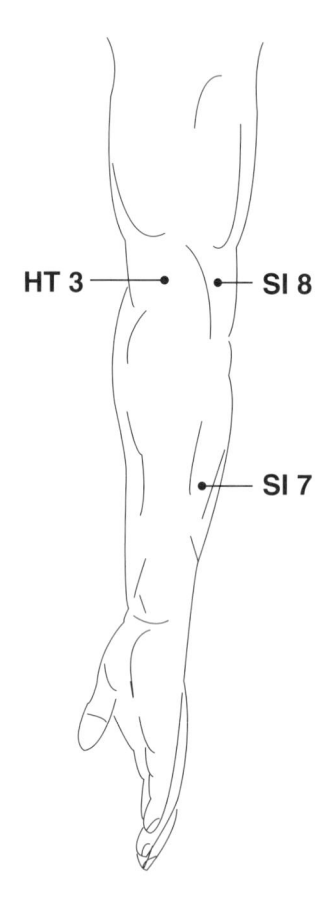

Fig. 16-8. Acupuncture Points in the Elbow and the Forearm
- Medial Surface View

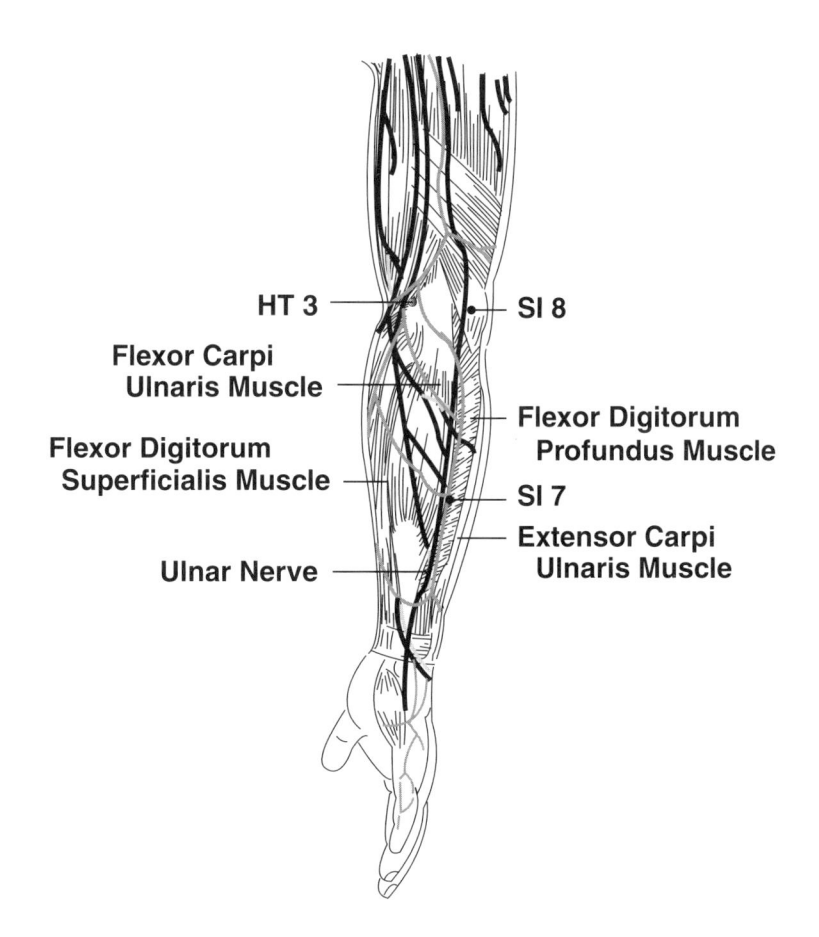

Fig. 16-9. Acupuncture Points in the Elbow and the Forearm
- Medial Superficial View

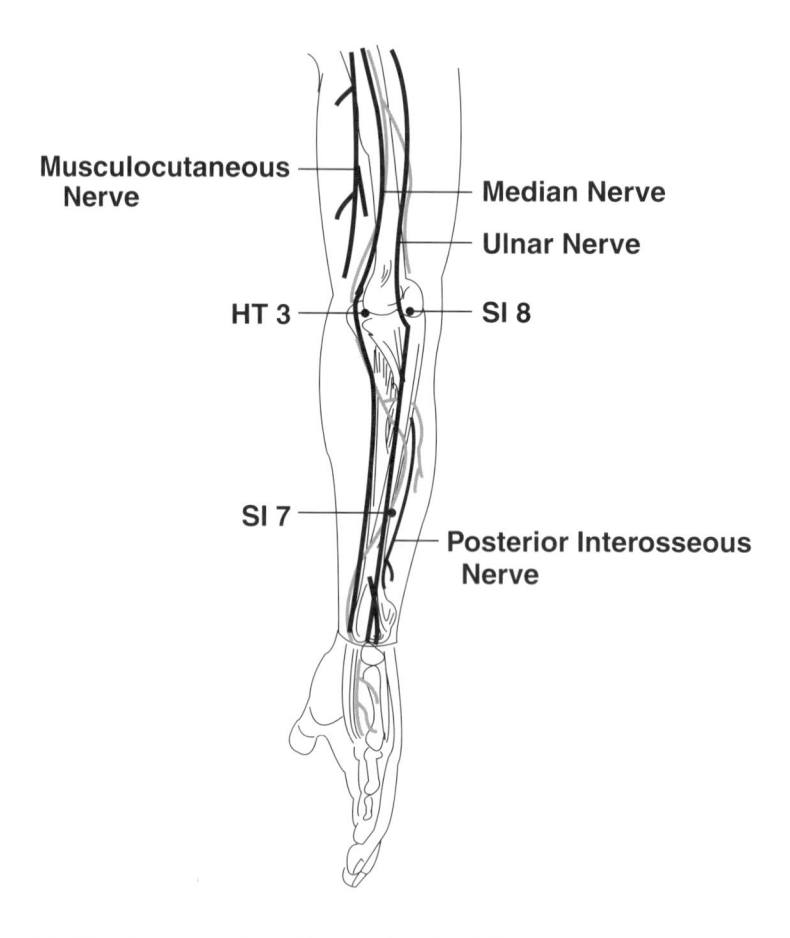

Fig. 16-10. Acupuncture Points in the Elbow and the Forearm
 - Medial Deep View

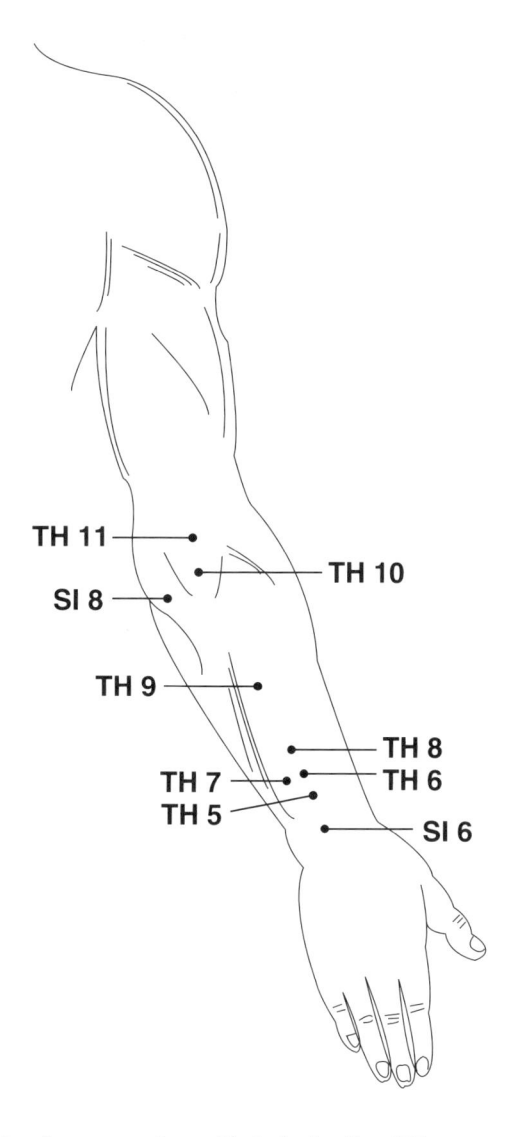

Fig. 16-11. Acupuncture Points in the Elbow and the Forearm
 - Posterior Surface View

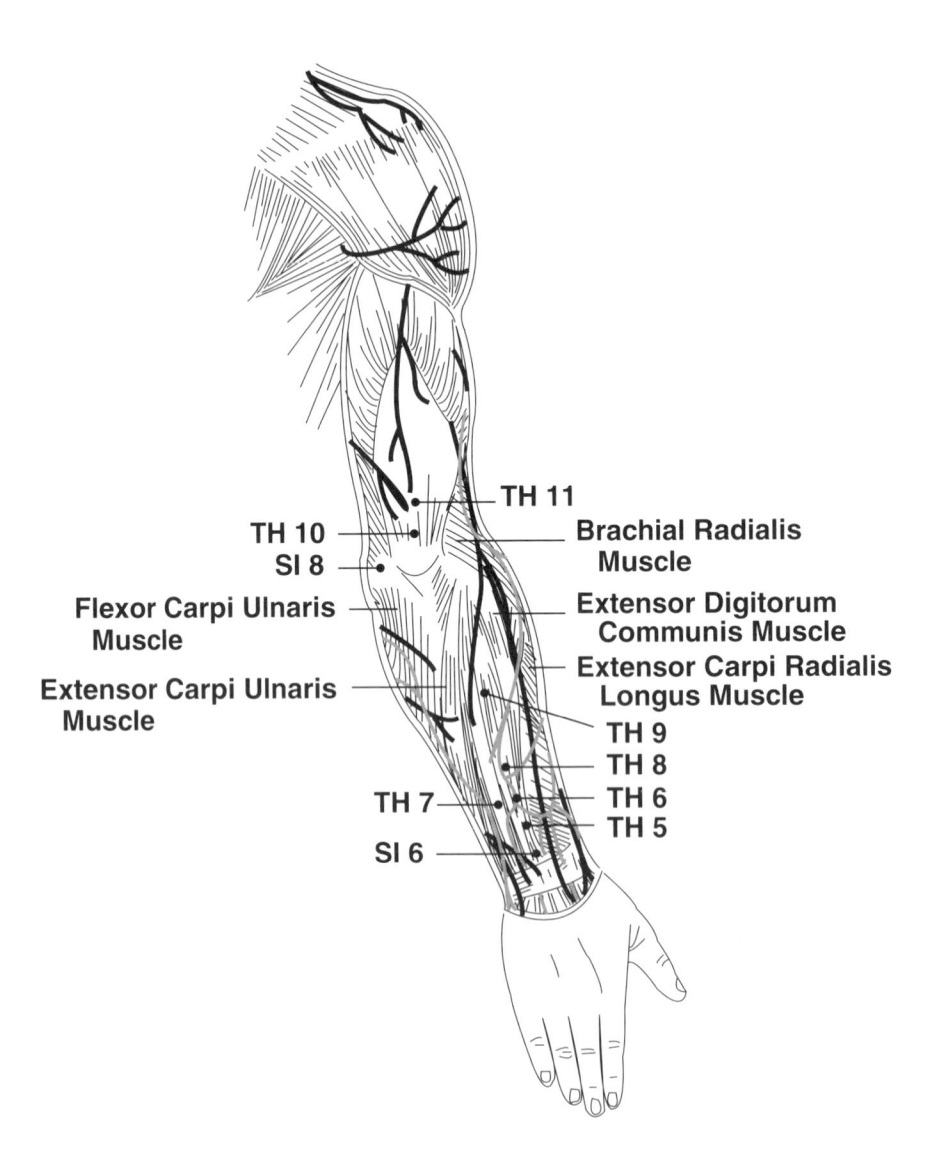

Fig. 16-12. Acupuncture Points in the Elbow and the Forearm
- Posterior Superficial View

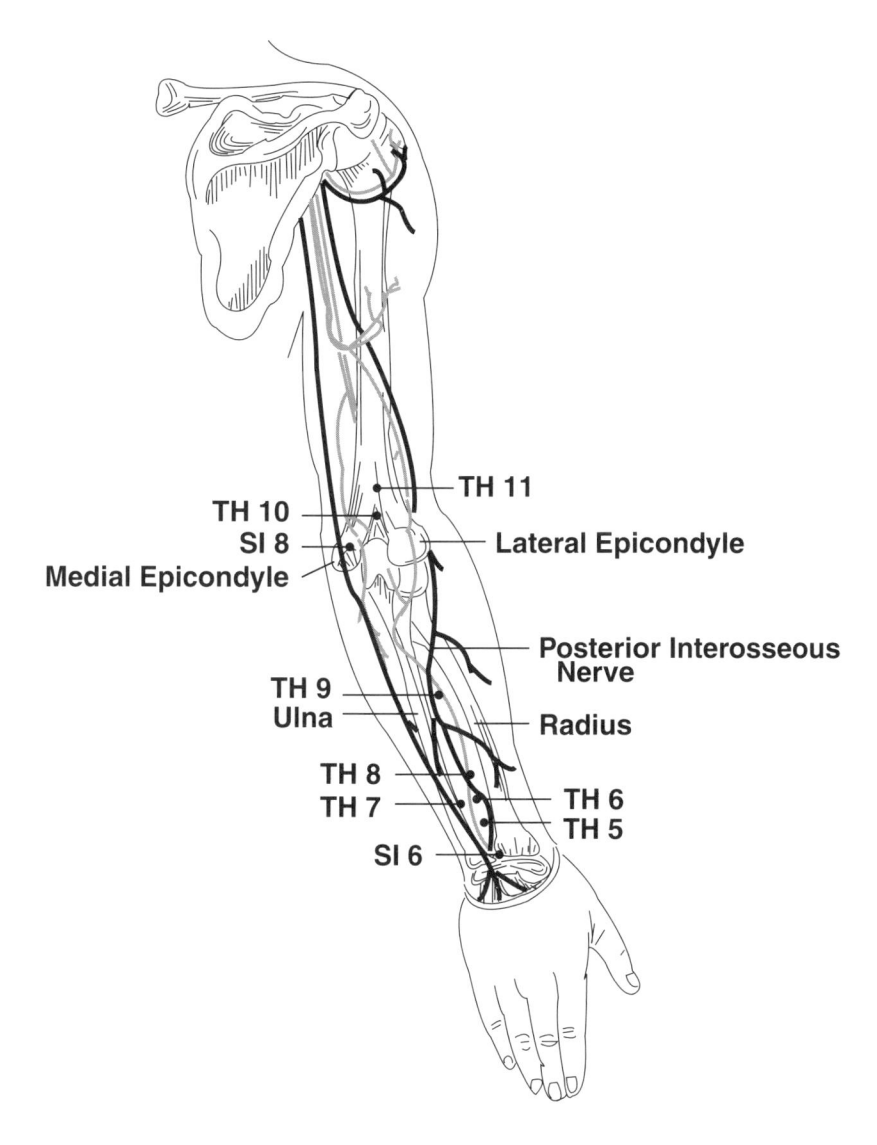

Fig. 16-13. Acupuncture Points in the Elbow and the Forearm
- Posterior Deep View

Nerve Stimulation in the Elbow

Table 16-2

	Name of Nerve	Acupuncture Point
Direct Stimulation to Elbow	elbow joint (intra-articular)	LU 5, PC 3
Peripheral Nerve	radial nerve	LU 5, LI 10, LI 11, TH 9, TH 8, TH 6, TH 5
	median nerve	PC 3, PC 4, PC 5, PC 6
	ulnar nerve	SI 7, SI 8, HT 3, HT 4, TH 7

Elbow and Forearm Muscles

Table 16-3

Muscle	Action	Innervation Peripheral Nerve	Innervation Spinal Segment	Acupuncture Point
Biceps Brachii	flexes and supinates forearm	musculocutaneous nerve	C 5, C 6	LU 3, LU 4, PC 2
Brachialis	flexes forearm	musculocutaneous nerve	C 5, C 6	LU 3, LU 4, PC 2
Triceps Brachii	extends forearm	radial nerve	C 6 - C 8	LI 11, TH 11, LU 5
Supinator	supinates forearm	radial nerve	C 5, C 6	LI 11, LU 5
Anconeus	extends forearm	radial nerve	C 7, C 8, T 1	LI 11, LU 5
Brachio-Radialis	flexes forearm	radial nerve	C 5, C 6	LI 10, LI 11, LI 12, TH 9, LU 5
Pronator Teres	pronates and flexes forearm	median nerve	C 6, C 7	PC 6, PC 5, PC 4, PC 3

Muscle	Action	Peripheral Nerve	Spinal Segment	Acupuncture Point
Pronator Quadratus	pronates forearm	medial nerve	C 7, C 8, T 1	PC 6, PC 5
Extensor Carpi Radialis Longus	extends and abducts hand	radial nerve	C 7, C 8	LI 10, LI 11, LI 12, TH 9, LU 5
Extensor Carpi Radialis Brevis	extends and abducts hand	radial nerve	C 7, C 8	LI 10, LI 11, LI 12, TH 9, LU 5
Extensor Digitorum Communis	extends wrist and fingers	radial nerve	C 7, C 8	LI 10, LI 11, TH 9, TH 5
Extensor Carpi Ulnaris	extends and adducts hand and 5th metacarpal	radial nerve	C 7, C 8	LI 10, LI 11, TH 9
Flexor Carpi Radialis	flexes and abducts hand	median nerve	C 6 - C 8	PC 5, PC 6
Palmaris Longus	flexes hand	median nerve	C 7, C 8, T 1	PC 5, PC 6
Flexor Digitorum Sublimis	flexes hand and fingers	median nerve	C 7, C 8, T 1	PC 6
Flexor Digitorum Profundus	flexes hand and fingers	median nerve	C 7, C 8, T 1	PC 6
Flexor Carpi Ulnaris	flexes and adducts hand	ulnar nerve	C 6 - C 8	HT 4, HT 5, HT 6, HT 7
Flexor Pollicis Longus	flexes thumb	median nerve	C 7, C 8, T 1	PC 6
Extensor Digiti Quinti	extends little finger	radial nerve	C 7, C 8	TH 7

Clinical Application

Osteoarthritis and Rheumatoid Arthritis of Elbow

- intra-articular points: LU 5, PC 3
- for rheumatoid arthritis, add immune mechanism points: LI 4, ST 36, BL 23, SP 10, SP 6 (see page 106)
- peripheral nerve stimulation for elbow joint: radial nerve – LI 11, median nerve – PC 3, ulnar nerve – SI 8

Ligamentous Strain of the Elbow

- LI 11, LU 5 for lateral collateral ligaments
- PC 3, HT 3 for medial collateral ligaments

Lateral Epicondylitis (Tennis Elbow)

- pain and tenderness over lateral epicondyle
- wrist extension with resistance gives rise to pain to lateral epicondyle
- LI 10, LI 11, LU 5, TH 9 for radial nerve proximal stimulation
- TH 5 for radial nerve distal stimulation

Strain of the Common Extensor Tendon

- attaching to lateral epicondyle at teno-osseous site
- extensor carpi radialis brevis tendon commonly involved
- best treated with a combination of LI 10 and LI 11

Tendinitis of Tendons Attaching to Lateral Epicondyle

- TH 8, TH 9 for extensor digitorum communis
- TH 9, TH 7 for extensor digiti quinti
- TH 9, TH 7 for extensor carpi ulnaris
- LI 10, LI 11 for extensor carpi radialis brevis
- LI 11, LU 5 for supinator
- LI 11, LU 5 for anconeus
- GB 34 or C 6 Spinal Nerve point for acupuncture mobilization, manipulation or exercises

Medial Epicondylitis (Golfer's Elbow)

- valgus stress of elbow resulting in periosteum inflammation
- possibly a lesion in common flexor tendon attaching to medial epicondlye
- painful resisted wrist flexion
- median nerve stimulation with PC 3 (proximal), PC 6 (distal)
- HT 3 helps pronator teres

Tendinitis of Tendons Attaching to Medial Epicondyle

- PC 3, HT 3 for pronator teres
- PC 5, PC 6 for pronator quadratus
- PC 5, PC 6 for palmaris longus
- PC 5, PC 6 for flexor carpi radialis
- PC 6 for flexor digitorum sublimus
- PC 6 for flexor digitorum profundus
- HT 4, HT 5 for flexor carpi ulnaris

Olecranon Bursitis

- swelling and inflammation of olecranon bursa
- excessive swelling may require aspiration
- TH 10 relieves pain and resolves inflammation

Tenosynovitis

- usually due to repetitive strain
- extensor carpi ulnaris tendon most commonly affected
- SI 6 in combination with TH 7
- TH 5, TH 6 for extensor carpi radialis longus and brevis

Radial Tunnel Syndrome

- radial nerve entrapment in a tunnel between extensor carpi radialis longus and brachioradialis muscles
- good prognosis for recovery with LI 11 and TH 5 without axonopathy
- severe radial entrapment may require surgical decompression

Chapter Seventeen

The Wrist and the Hand

Acupuncture Meridians and Points in the Wrist and the Hand

There are six meridians crossing the wrist and the hand:

Table 17-1

Meridian	Acupuncture Point	Location
Large Intestine Meridian (LI)	LI 5	radial side of wrist in depression between tendons of extensor pollicis brevis and extensor pollicis longus
	LI 4	between 1st and 2nd metacarpal bones at midpoint of 2nd metacarpal bone
	LI 3	on radial side of index finger, proximal to MCP joint
	LI 2	on radial side of index finger, distal to MCP joint
	LI 1	on radial side of index finger, 0.1 cun to corner of nail
Triple Heater Meridian (TH)	TH 4	at junction of ulna and carpal bones, in depression lateral to extensor digitorum communis
	TH 3	on dorsum of hand between 4th and 5th metacarpal bones, proximal to MCP joint
	TH 2	between ring and little fingers, proximal to margin of web
	TH 1	on ulnar side of 4th finger, 0.1 cun to corner of nail

Meridian	Acupuncture Point	Location
Small Intestine Meridian (SI)	SI 5	on ulnar side of wrist, between ulnar styloid process and carpal bone
	SI 4	on ulnar side of wrist, between 5th metacarpal bone and carpal bone
	SI 3	on ulnar side of metacarpal bone, proximal to MCP joint
	SI 2	on ulnar side of little finger, distal to MCP joint
	SI 1	on ulnar side of little finger, 0.1 cun to corner of nail
Lung Meridian (LU)	LU 7	on radial side of radial styloid process, 1.5 cun proximal to wrist crease
	LU 8	on radial aspect of radial styloid process, 0.5 cun distal to wrist crease
	LU 9	on volar wrist crease, on radial side of radial artery
	LU 10	on thenar eminence, on ulnar side of metacarpal bone at midpoint of metacarpal bone
	LU 11	on radial side of thumb, 0.1 cun to corner of nail
Pericardium Meridian (PC)	PC 7	midpoint on palmar wrist crease, between palmary longus and flexor carpi radialis
	PC 8	between 2nd and 3rd metacarpal bones, proximal to MCP joint
	PC 9	at tip of middle finger
Heart Meridian (HT)	HT 7	on volar wrist crease, on radial side of flexor carpi ulnaris
	HT 8	between 4th and 5th metacarpal bones proximal to MCP joint
	HT 9	on radial side of little finger, 0.1 cun to corner of nail

Neuro-Anatomical Analysis of LI 4

Stimulation of peripheral nerves:	• radial nerve (skin) • ulnar nerve (1st interosseous and pollicis adductor brevis muscles) • median nerve (thenar muscles)
Impulse to spinal segments:	C 4 to C 8 – T 1, covering the whole brachial plexus
Stimulation of sympathetic nerve system:	rich sympathetic nerve fibres in double palmar arterial arches of hand

Extra-Meridian Points

Table 17-2

Point	Location
Shixuan	at tip of all fingers
Baxie	on dorsum of hand, in web between fingers, eight points in all
Louzhen	on dorsum of hand, between 2nd and 3rd metacarpal bones, 0.5 cun proximal to metacarpal joint
Lumbago # 1	on dorsum of hand, midpoint between 2nd and 3rd metacarpal bones
Lumbago # 2	on dorsum of hand, midpoint between 4th and 5th metacarpal bones

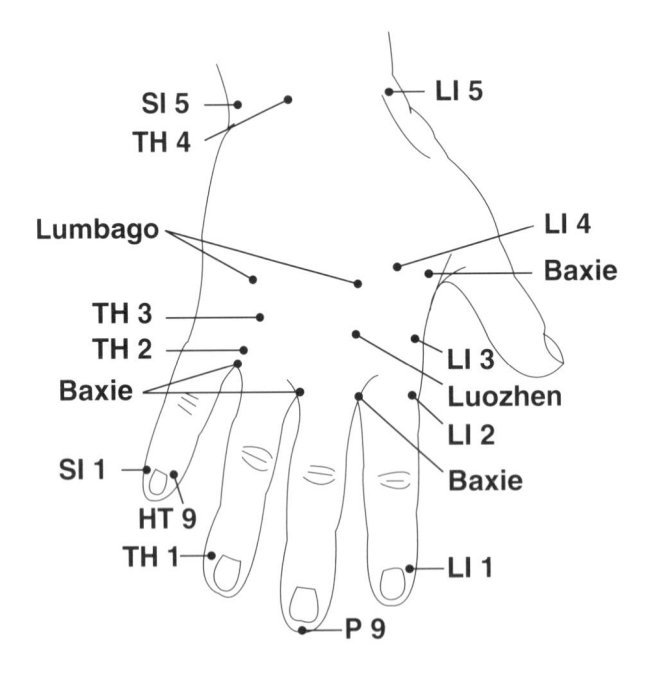

Fig. 17-1. Acupuncture Points in the Wrist and the Hand
- Dorsal Surface View

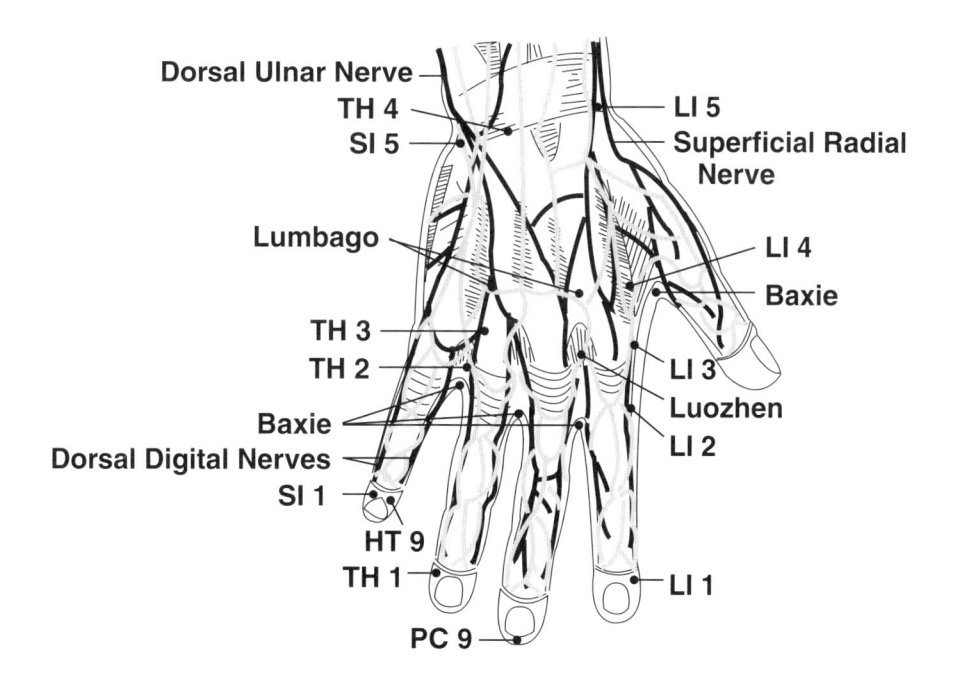

Fig. 17-2. Acupuncture Points in the Wrist and the Hand
 - Dorsal Superficial View

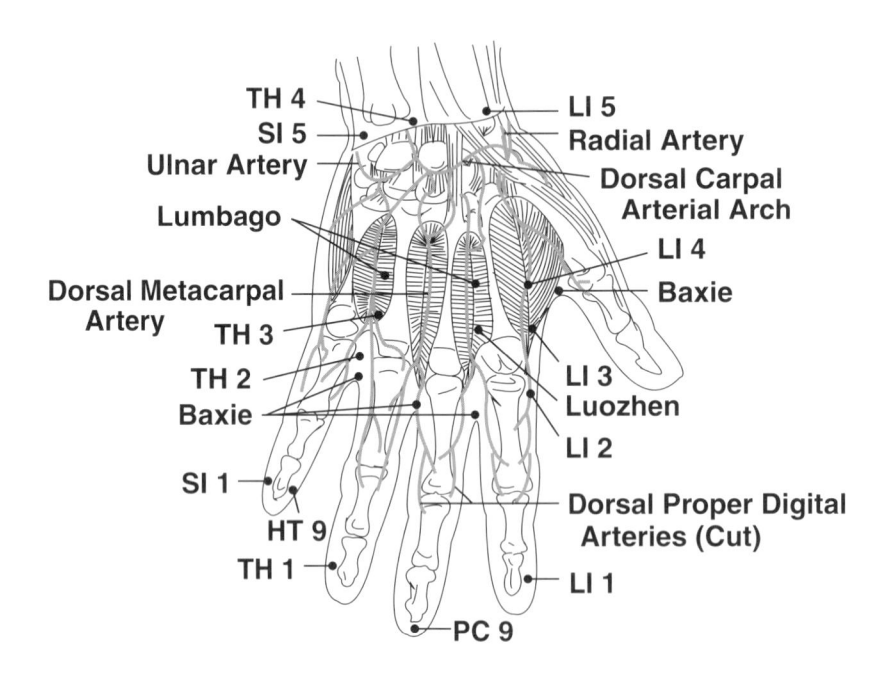

Fig. 17-3. Acupuncture Points in the Wrist and the Hand
 - Dorsal Deep View

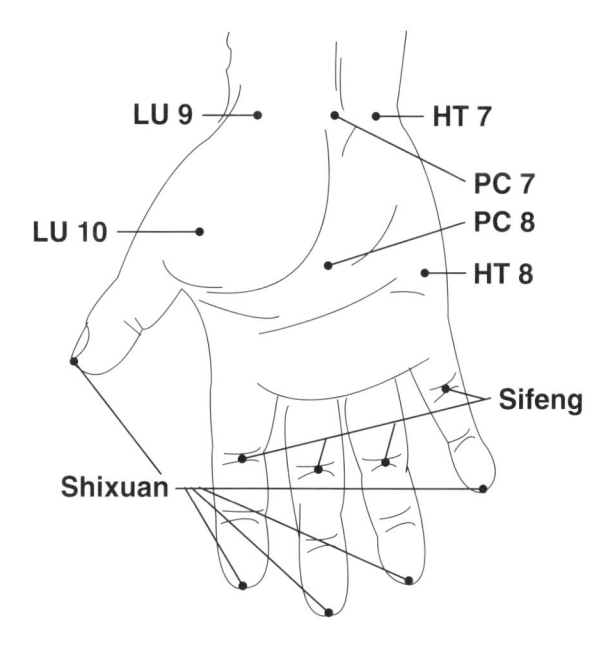

Fig. 17-4. Acupuncture Points in the Wrist and the Hand
 - Palmar Surface View

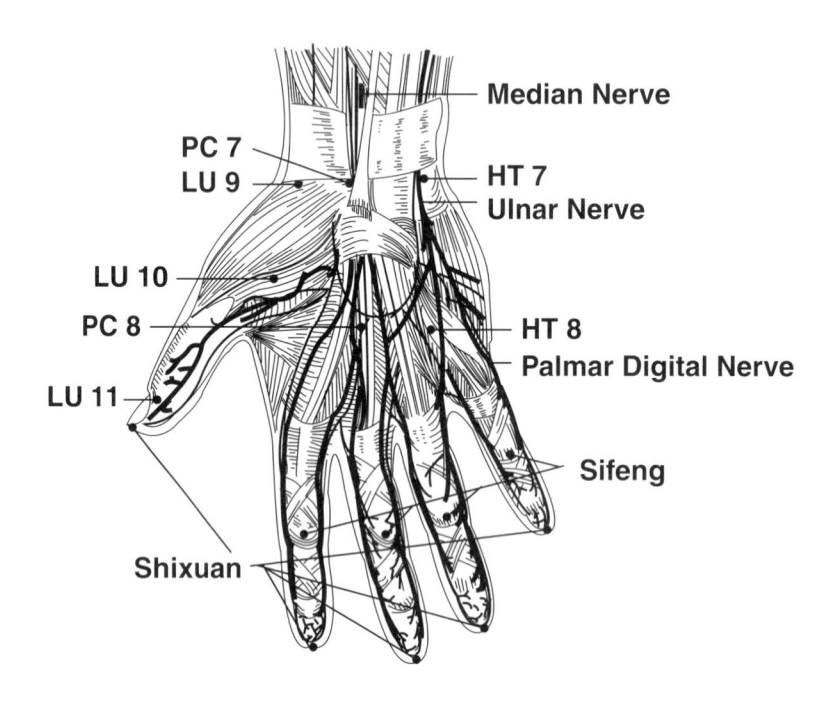

Fig. 17-5. Acupuncture Points in the Wrist and the Hand
 - Palmar Superficial View

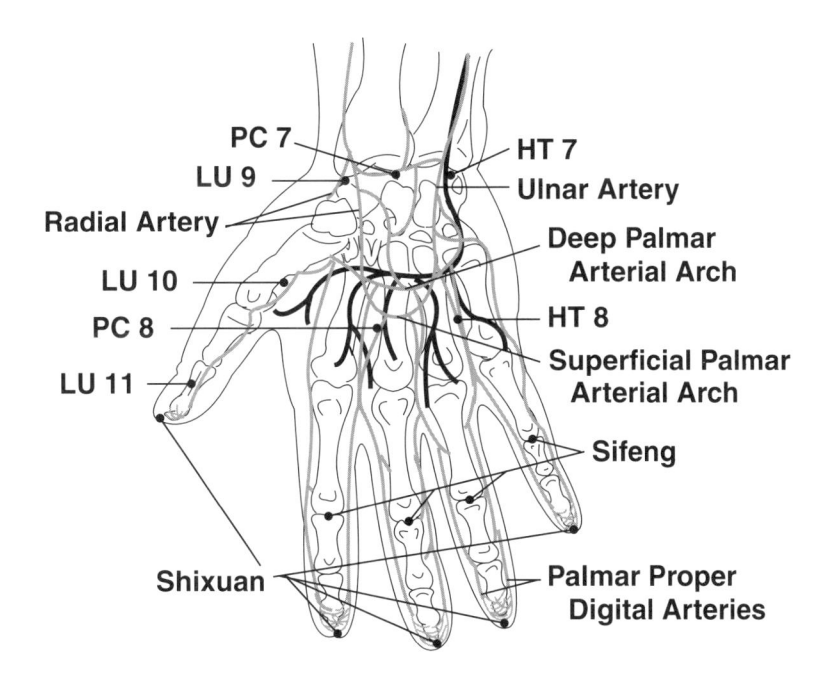

Fig. 17-6. Acupuncture Points in the Wrist and the Hand
 - Palmar Deep View

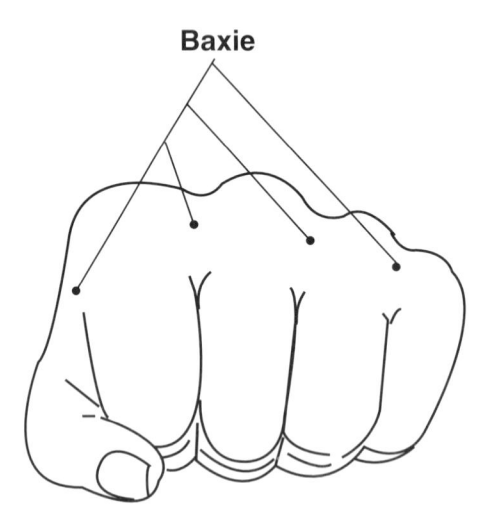

Fig. 17-7. Extra-Meridian Point - Baxie

Nerve Stimulation in the Wrist and the Hand

Table 17-3

	Name of Nerve	Acupuncture Point
Direct Stimulation to Wrist	wrist joint (intra-articular)	TH 4, PC 7
Peripheral Nerve in Wrist	radial nerve	LI 5, LU 9
	median nerve	PC 7
	ulnar nerve	SI 5, HT 7
Peripheral Nerve in Hand	radial nerve	LI 4, LI 3, L 2, L 1, TH 3, TH 2, TH 1
	median nerve	LU 10, LU 11, PC 8, PC 9
	ulnar nerve	HT 8, HT 9, SI 4, SI 3, SI 2, SI 1

Hand Muscles

Table 17-4

Muscle	Action	Innervation Peripheral Nerve	Spinal Segment	Acupuncture Point
Abductor Pollicis Longus	abducts thumb	radial nerve	C 6 - C 8	LI 5
Extensor Pollicis Brevis	extends thumb and abducts 1st metacarpal	radial nerve	C 6 - C 8	LI 5
Abductor Pollicis Brevis	abducts thumb, flexes 1st and extends 2nd phalanx	median nerve	C 6 - C 8, T 1	LU 10
Flexor Pollicis Brevis	flexes and adducts thumb	median nerve	C 6 - C 8, T 1	LU 10
Opponens Pollicis	flexes, adducts and rotates thumb medially	median nerve	C 6 - C 8, T 1	LU 10
Adductor Pollicis	adducts and flexes thumb	ulnar nerve	C 8, T 1	LI 4
Abductor Digiti Quinti	abducts little finger, flexes 1st phalanx of little finger	ulnar nerve	C 8, T 1	SI 3
Opponens Digiti Quinti	flexes and adducts little finger	ulnar nerve	C 8, T 1	SI 3
Flexor Digiti Quinti	flexes 1st phalanx of little finger	ulnar nerve	C 8, T 1	SI 3

Clinical Application

Osteoarthritis or Rheumatoid Arthritis in the Wrist

- intra-articular points PC 7, TH 4

- peripheral nerve stimulation for wrist joint: LI 5, LU 9 for radial nerve; SI 5, HT 7 for ulnar nerve; PC 7 for median nerve

- for rheumatoid arthritis, add immune mechanism points: LI 4, ST 36, BL 23, SP 10, SP 6 (see page 106)

Collateral Ligamentous Strain

- acute traumatic strain or chronic repetitive strain

- peripheral nerve stimulation: LI 5, LU 9 for radial nerve; SI 5, HT 7 for ulnar nerve; PC 7 for median nerve

Carpal Tunnel Syndrome

- compression of median nerve in carpal tunnel

- inflammatory mechanism in early stage

- Wallerian degeneration and intraneural fibrosis in late stage

- best treated with acupuncture points: PC 7, PC 8

- better result with LI 4 in combination (contra-indicated in pregnancy)

- severe compression may require surgical decompression

de Quervain's Tenosynovitis

- abductor pollicis longus and extensor pollicis brevis tendons involved
- inflammation of synovial sheath resulting in stenosing tenosynovitis
- occasionally a ganglion is associated
- LI 4, LI 5 relieve pain and inflammation
- ganglion may disappear after multiple insertions of acupuncture needle to midpoint of ganglion

Osteoarthritis or Rheumatoid Arthritis of Hand and Fingers

- peripheral nerve stimulation of digital nerve using extra-meridian point, Baxie
- LI 3 may stimulate four palmar digital nerves simultaneously
- LI 4 normalizes sympathetic dysfunctions
- extra-meridian points, Sifeng, particularly for proximal interphalangeal joints
- for rheumatoid arthritis, add immune mechanism points: LI 4, ST 36, BL 23, SP 10, SP 6 (see page 106)

Trigger Finger

- tendons commonly involved: flexor pollicis longus, middle or ring finger flexor tendons
- nodule formation and snapping phenomenon during flexion and re-extension
- extra-meridian points: Sifeng, to flexor surface of PIP joint
- other points: LU 10 for thumb; PC 8 for middle or ring finger

Chapter Eighteen

The Hip

Acupuncture Meridians and Points in the Hip

There are five meridians crossing the hip:

Table 18-1

Meridian	Acupuncture Point	Location
Stomach Meridian (ST)	ST 31	inferior to anterior superior iliac spine, between sartorius and tensor fascia lata muscles
	ST 32	in rectus femoris muscle, 6 cun superior to upper margin of patella
Gall Bladder Meridian (GB)	GB 27	medial to anterior superior iliac spine
	GB 28	0.5 cun inferior and slightly medial to GB 27
	GB 29	midpoint between anterior superior iliac spine and greater trochanter
	GB 30	one-third of distance from greater trochanter to hiatus sacralis
	GB 31	on lateral aspect of thigh, 7 cun superior to knee joint line
Urinary Bladder Meridian (BL)	BL 36	midpoint of transverse gluteal fold
	BL 37	6 cun distal to BL 36
Spleen Meridian (SP)	SP 12	superior to midpoint of inguinal ligament, lateral to femoral artery
	SP 13	1 cun superior to SP 12
Liver Meridian (LR)	LR 10	2 cun distal to pubic ramus, lateral to adductor longus
	LR 11	1 cun distal to pubic ramus, lateral to adductor longus

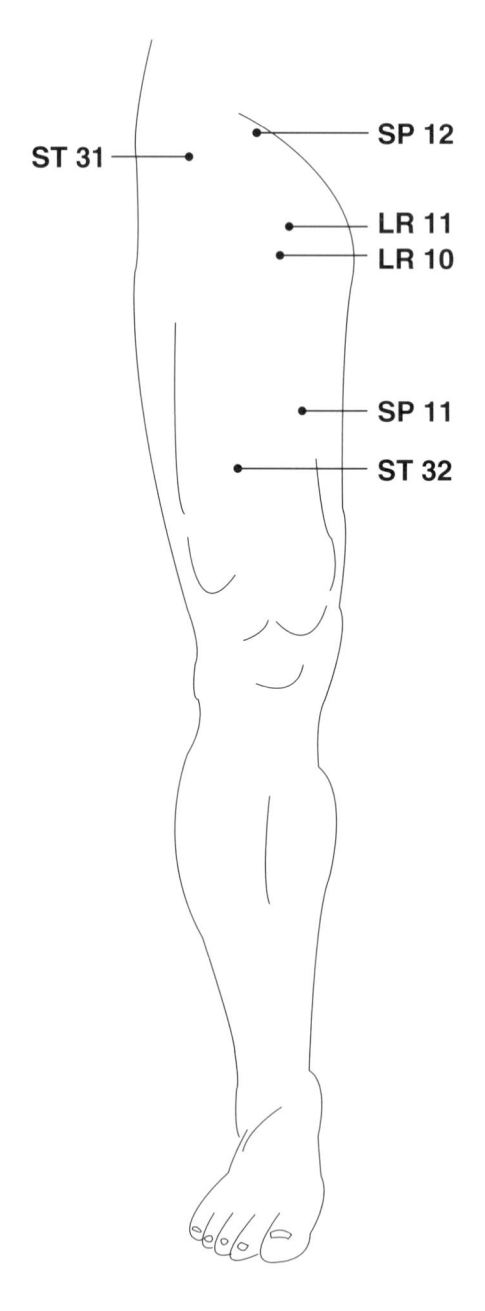

Fig. 18-1. Acupuncture Points in the Hip
- Anterior Surface View

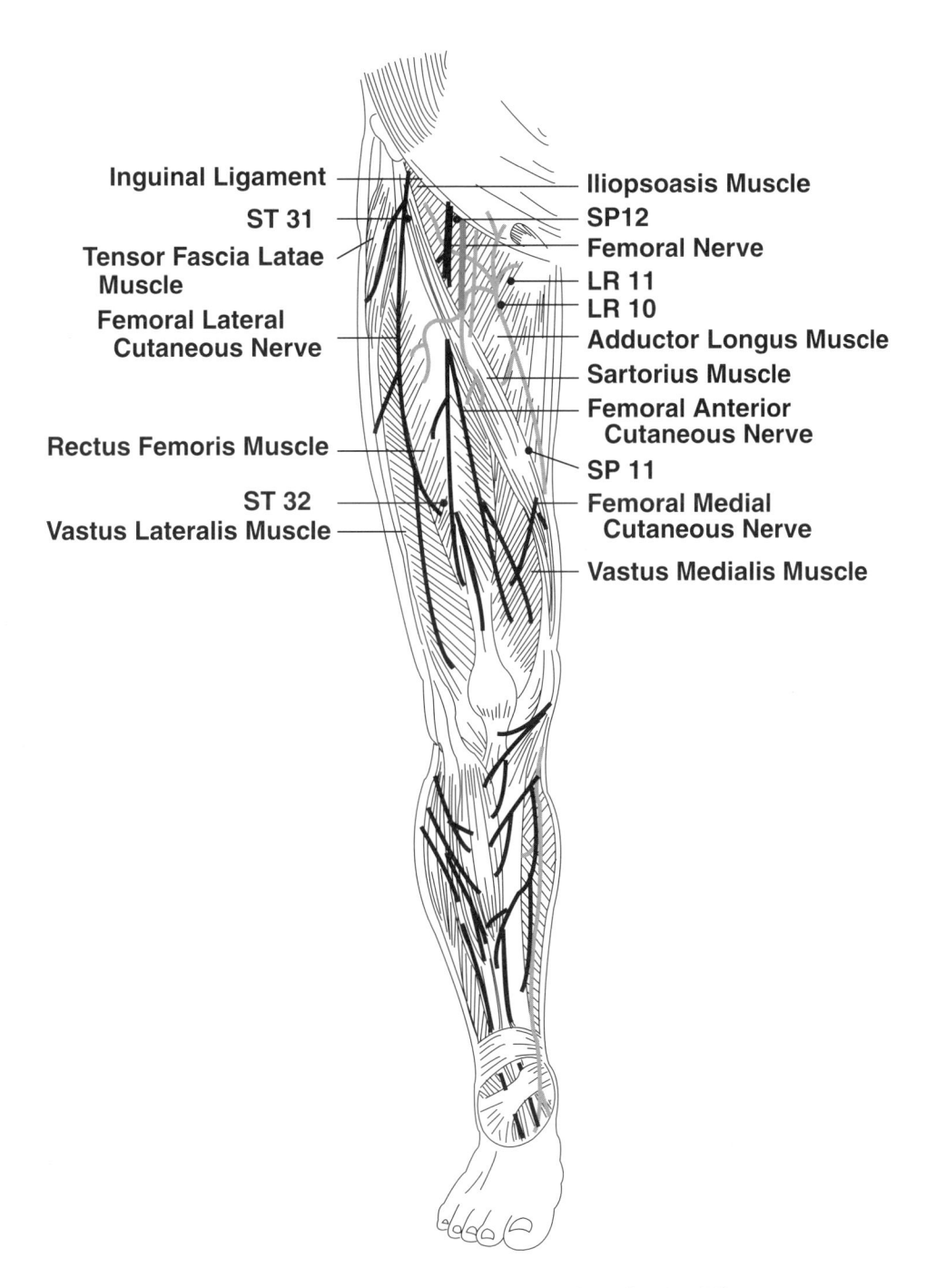

Fig. 18-2. Acupuncture Points in the Hip
- Anterior Superficial View

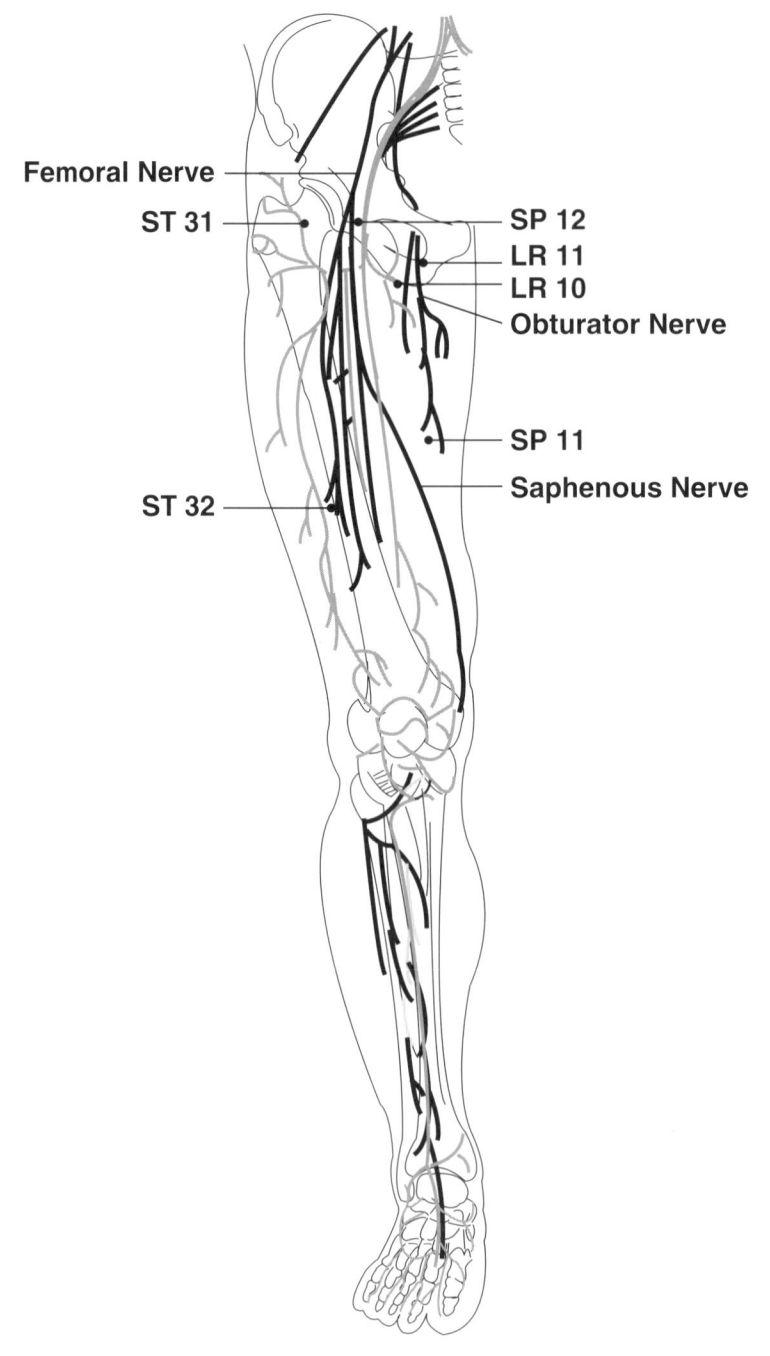

Fig. 18-3. Acupuncture Points in the Hip
- Anterior Deep View

GB 29
GB 30

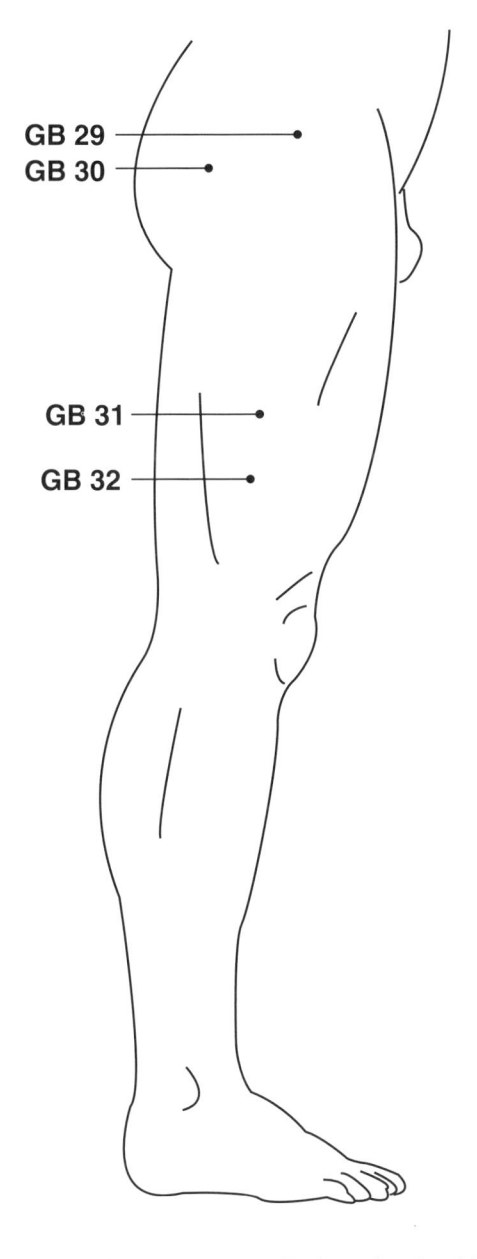

GB 31
GB 32

**Fig. 18-4. Acupuncture Points in the Hip
- Lateral Surface View**

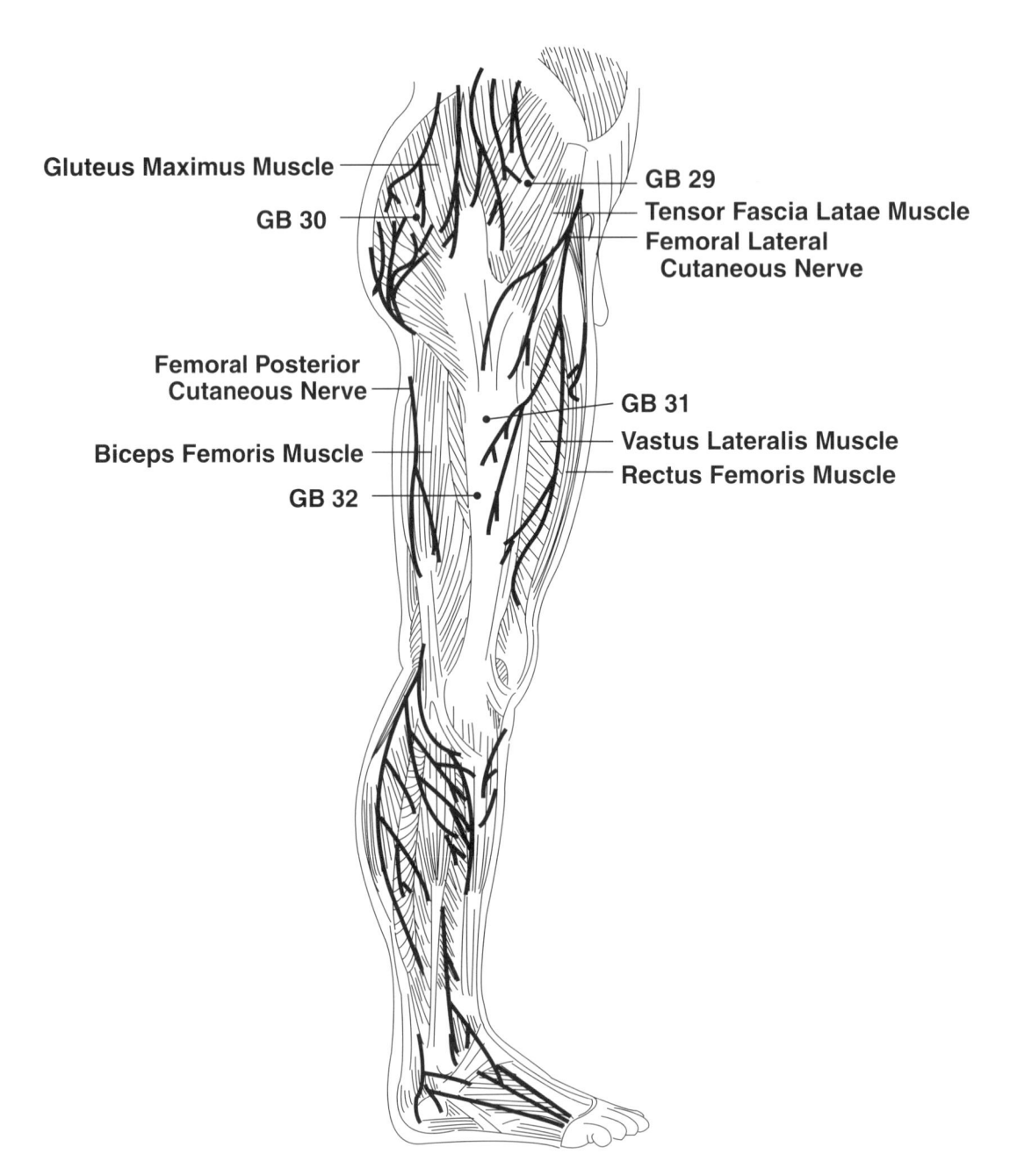

Fig. 18-5. Acupuncture Points in the Hip
- Lateral Superficial View

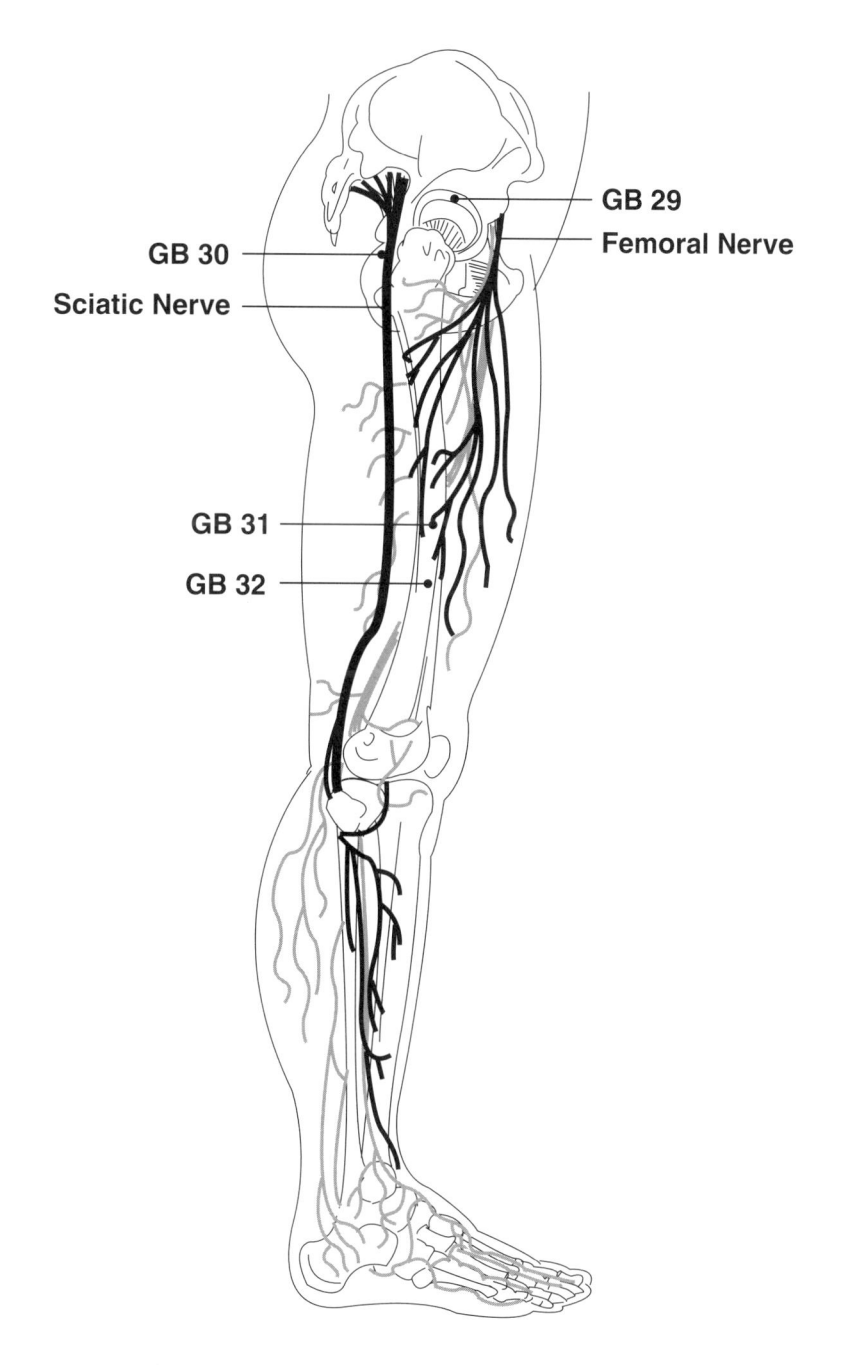

Fig. 18-6. Acupuncture Points in the Hip
- Lateral Deep View

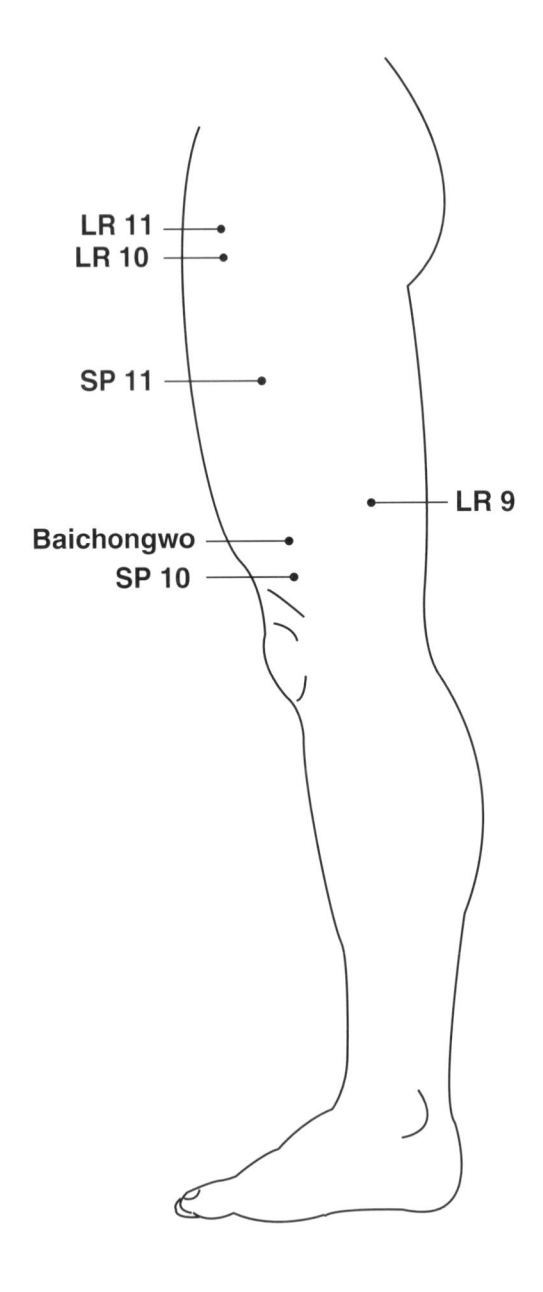

Fig. 18-7. Acupuncture Points in the Hip
- Medial Surface View

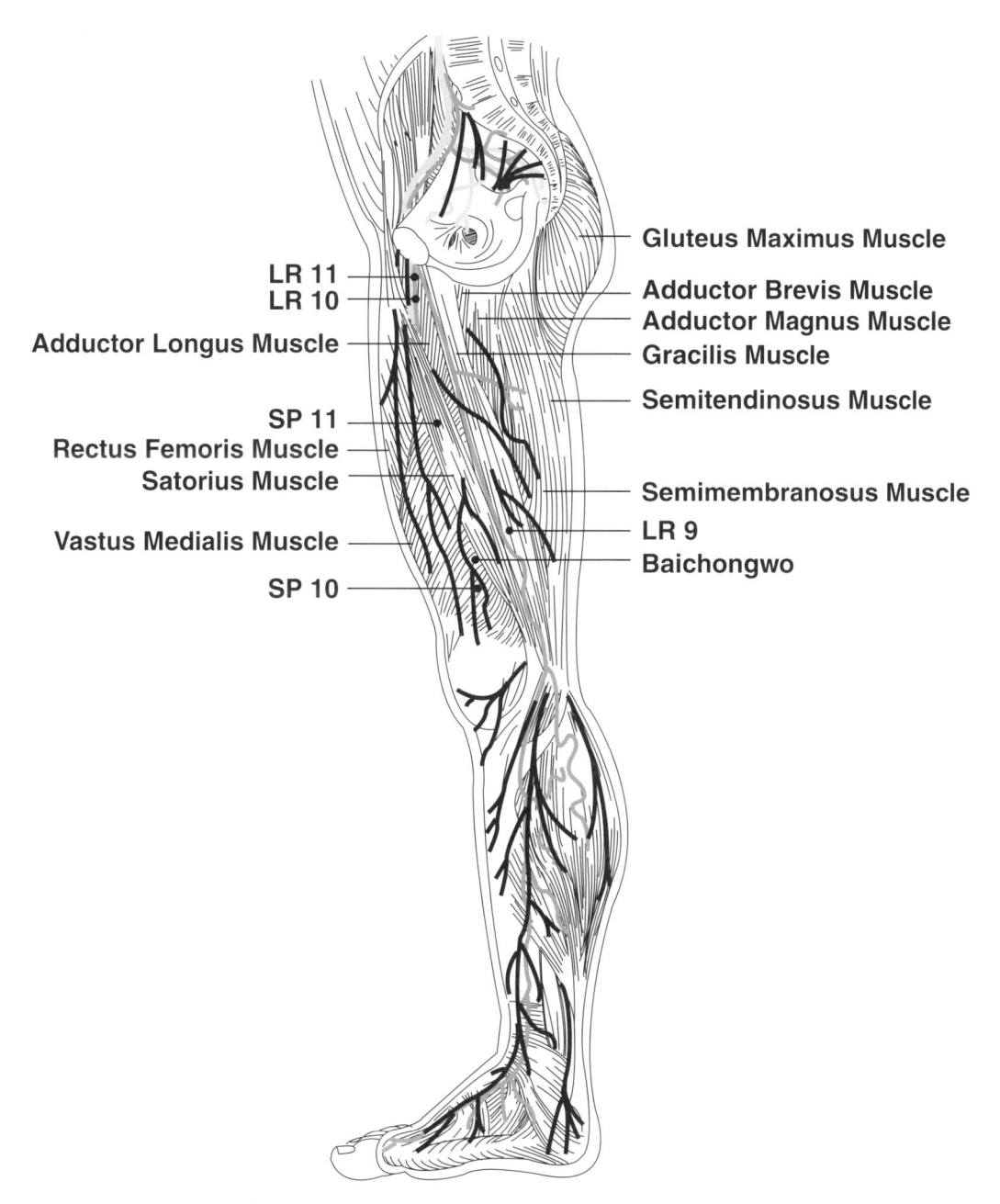

Fig. 18-8. Acupuncture Points in the Hip
- Medial Superficial View

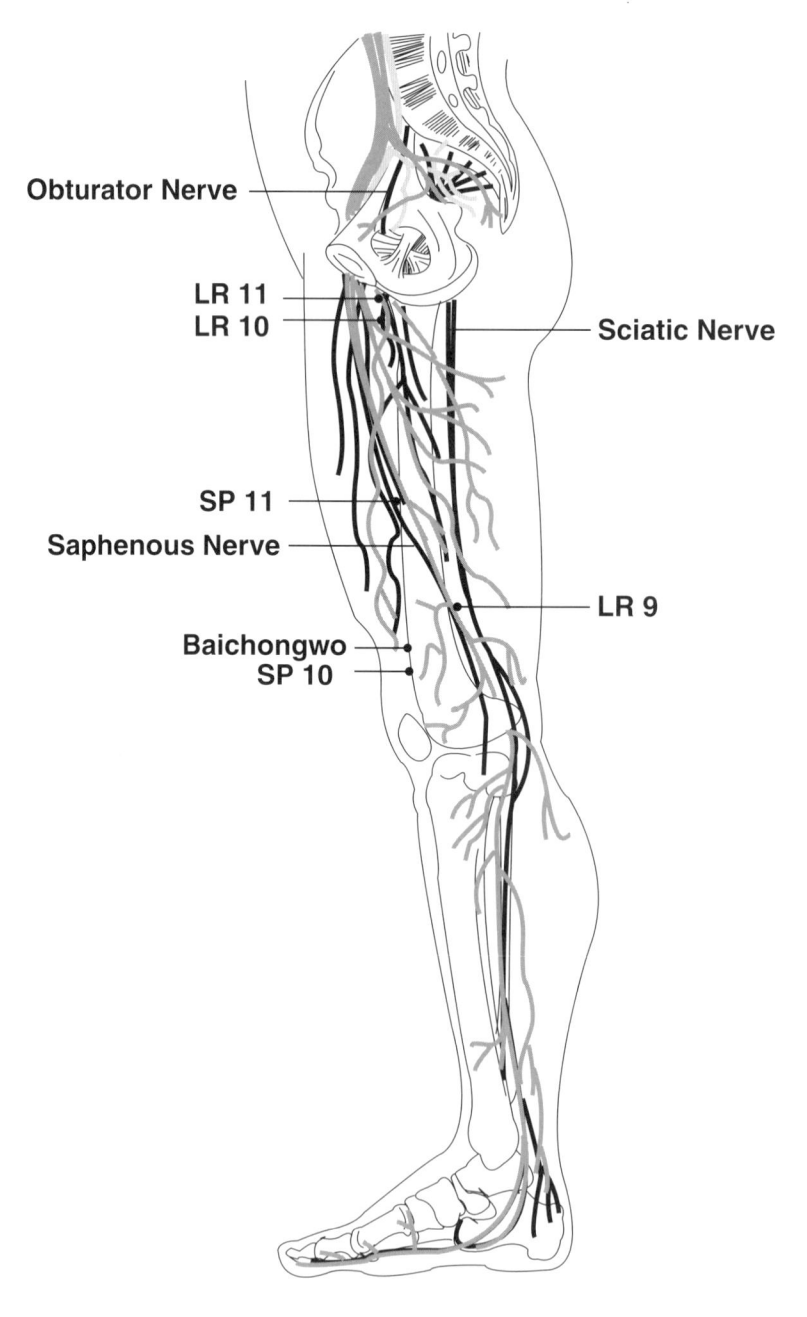

Fig. 18-9. Acupuncture Points in the Hip
- Medial Deep View

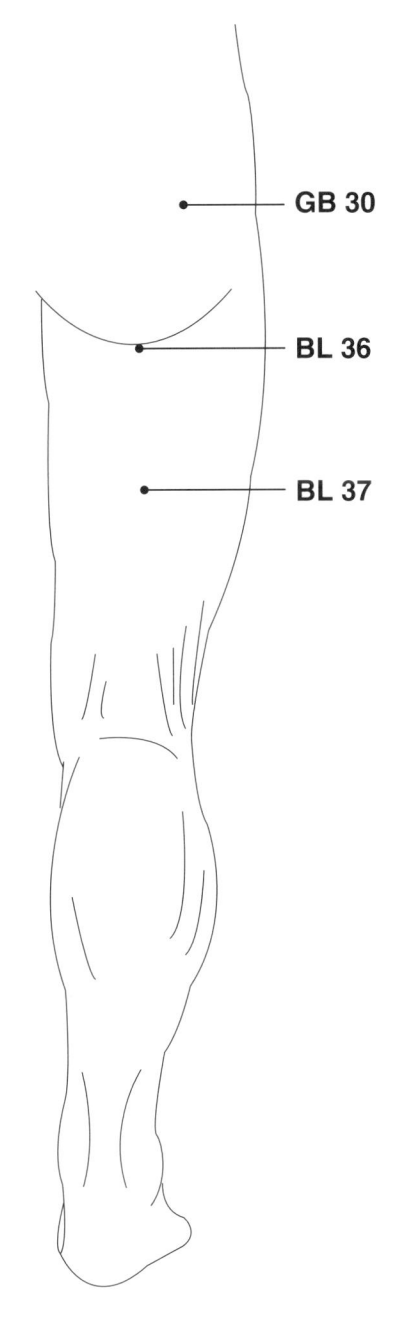

Fig. 18-10. Acupuncture Points in the Hip
- Posterior Surface View

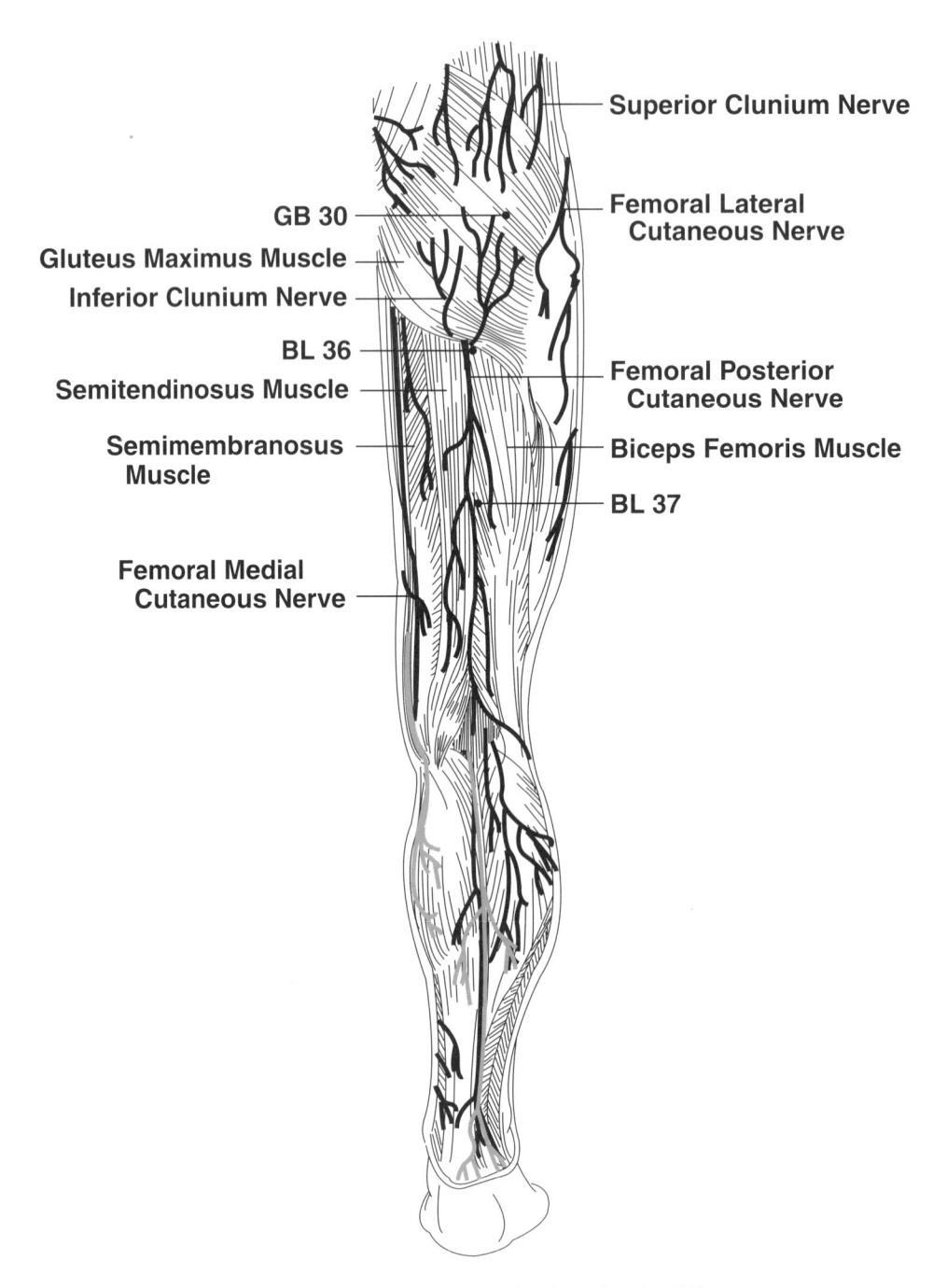

Fig. 18-11. Acupuncture Points in the Hip
- Posterior Superficial View

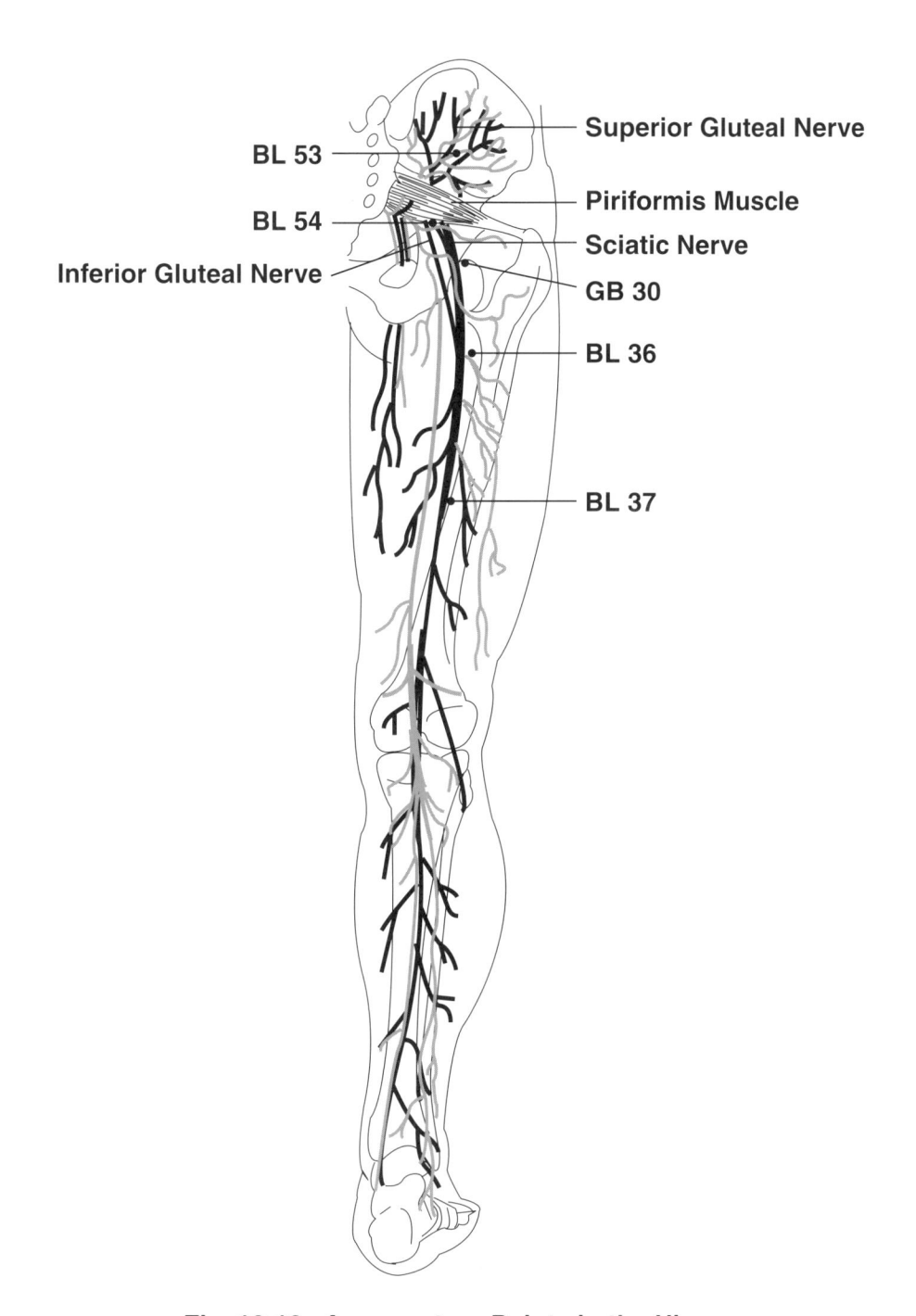

Fig. 18-12. Acupuncture Points in the Hip
- Posterior Deep View

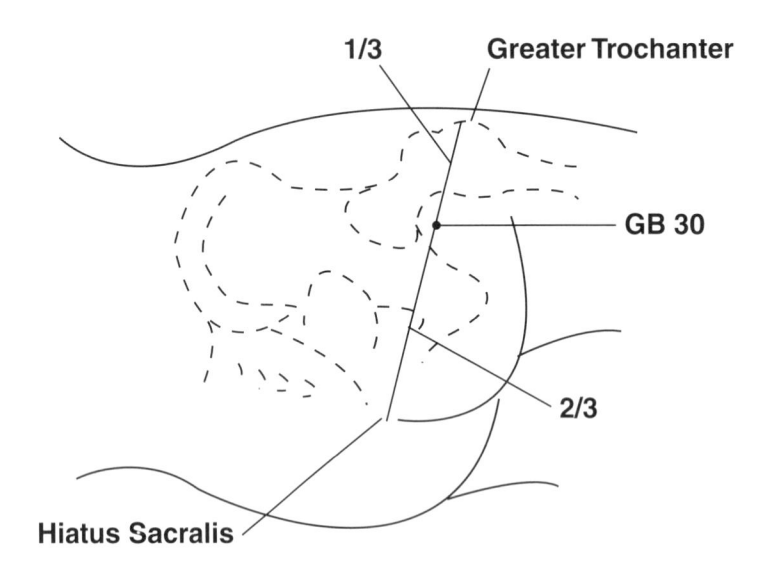

Fig. 18-13. Acupuncture Point GB 30

Nerve Stimulation in the Hip

Table 18-2

	Name of Nerve	Acupuncture Point
Direct Stimulation to the Hip	hip joint (intra-articular)	GB 29
Peripheral Nerve	sciatic nerve	GB 30, BL 36, BL 37
	femoral nerve	SP 12, SP 13
	obturator nerve	LR 10, LR 11
	superior gluteal nerve	BL 53
	inferior gluteal nerve	BL 54
Neuro-Plexus	sacral plexus	BL 54

Hip Muscles

Table 18-3

Muscle	Action	Peripheral Nerve	Spinal Segment	Acupuncture Point
Iliopsoas	flexes thigh, adducts and rotates thigh medially	femoral nerve	L 1 - L 3	SP 12
Sartorius	flexes thigh and rotates thigh laterally	femoral nerve	L 1 - L 3	SP 12
Rectus Femoris	flexes thigh	femoral nerve	L 2 - L 4	SP 12, ST 32
Gluteus Maximus	extends thigh, rotates thigh laterally	inferior gluteal nerve	L 5, S 1, S 2	BL 54
Gluteus Medius	abducts thigh, rotates thigh	superior gluteal nerve	L 4, L 5, S 1	BL 53
Gluteus Minimus	abducts and rotates thigh	superior gluteal nerve	L 4, L 5, S 1	BL 53

Muscle	Action	Peripheral Nerve	Spinal Segment	Acupuncture Point
Biceps Femoris	extends and adducts thigh	sciatic nerve	L 5, S 1, S 2	GB 30, BL 36, BL 37
Semitendinosus	extends and adducts thigh; rotates thigh medially	sciatic nerve	L 5, S 1, S 2	GB 30, BL 36, BL 37
Semimembranosus	extends and adducts thigh; rotates thigh medially	sciatic nerve	L 5, S 1, S 2	GB 30, BL 36, BL 37
Piriformis	extends, abducts and rotates thigh laterally	S 1, S 2 spinal nerves	S 1, S 2	BL 31, BL 32, BL 27, BL 28
Obturator Externus	rotates thigh laterally	obturator nerve	L 3, L 4	LR 10, LR 11
Obturator Internus	rotates thigh laterally	L 5, S 1 spinal nerves	L 5, S 1	BL 26, BL 27, BL 31
Gemelli	rotates thigh laterally	L 5, S 1 spinal nerves	L 5, S 1	BL 26, BL 27, BL 31
Quadratus Femoris	rotates thigh laterally	L 5, S 1 spinal nerves	L 5, S 1	BL 26, BL 27, BL 31
Pectineus	flexes and adducts thigh	femoral nerve	L 2, L 3	SP 12
Adductus Longus	adducts, flexes and rotates thigh laterally	obturator nerve	L 2, L 3	LR 10, LR 11
Adductus Brevis	adducts thigh	obturator nerve	L 2 - L 4	LR 10, LR 11

Muscle	Action	Peripheral Nerve	Spinal Segment	Acupuncture Point
Adductus Magnus	adducts thigh, assists in flexion, extension and lateral rotation	obturator nerve and sciatic nerve	L 4, L 5, S 1	GB 30, LR 10, LR 11
Tensor Fascia Lata	flexes, abducts and rotates thigh medially	superior gluteal nerve	L 4, L 5	BL 53, GB 31, GB 32
Gracilis	adducts and rotates thigh medially	obturator nerve	L 2, L 3	LR 10, LR 11

Clinical Application

Psoas Bursitis

- psoas bursa is largest single bursa in the body
- either due to direct trauma or overuse activity
- SP 12 stimulates femoral nerve
- ST 31 and ST 32 provide muscle relaxation

Gluteal and Trochanteric Bursitis

- due to either direct trauma or overuse activity
- may be associated with a tight iliotibial band
- tenderness over greater trochanter
- GB 29, GB 30, GB 31 relieve pain and swelling

Ischial Bursitis

- ischial bursa of gluteus maximus
- increase of pain on prolonged sitting
- BL 36, BL 37 stimulate sciatic nerve
- BL 54 stimulates inferior gluteal nerve

Osteoarthritis or Rheumatoid Arthritis of Hip Joint

- intra-articular point of hip joint: GB 29
- peripheral nerve stimulation for hip joint: posteriorly, GB 30; anteriorly, SP 12; medially, LR 10, LR 11
- for rheumatoid arthritis, add immune mechanism points, LI 4, ST 36, BL 23, SP 10, SP 6 (see page 106)

Hip Ligamentous Strain

- occasionally trapped ligamentum teres
- peripheral nerve stimulation: posteriorly, GB 30; anteriorly, SP 12

Rider's Strain

- adductus longus most commonly involved
- obturator nerve stimulation by LR 10 and LR 11

Hamstring Strain

- partial rupture and hematoma may occur
- pain localized inferior to ischial tuberosity
- pain aggravated by up-hill walking or running
- BL 36, BL 37 stimulate sciatic nerve

Hip Abductor Strain

- BL 53 stimulates superior gluteal nerve
- GB 31, GB 32 stimulate tensor fascia lata muscle (iliotibial band)
- GB 29 directly stimulates abductor muscles, tensor fascia lata, gluteus medius and minimus

Quadriceps Strain

- direct trauma may be responsible
- partial rupture or hematoma may occur
- SP 12 stimulates femoral nerve
- ST 32 stimulates quadriceps muscles

Chapter Nineteen

The Knee and the Leg

Acupuncture Meridians and Points in the Knee and the Leg

There are six meridians crossing the knee and leg:

Table 19-1

Meridian	Acupuncture Point	Location
Stomach Meridian (ST)	ST 32	in rectus femoris muscle, 6 cun superior to upper margin of patella
	ST 33	in vastus lateralis muscle, 3 cun superior to upper margin of patella
	ST 34	in vastus lateralis muscle, 2 cun superior to upper margin of patella
	ST 35	lateral to infrapatellar tendon (intra-articular)
	ST 36	3 cun inferior to lower margin of patella, 1 cun lateral to crest of tibia
Gall Bladder Meridian (GB)	GB 33	in depression between biceps femoris tendon and lateral condyle of femur
	GB 34	in depression anterior and inferior to head of fibula
Urinary Bladder Meridian (BL)	BL 38	1 cun superior to BL 39
	BL 39	on popliteal crease, medial to biceps femoris tendon
	BL 40	on popliteal crease, midpoint of popliteal fossa
Spleen Meridian (SP)	SP 9	posterior to tibia, on lower border of tibia medial condyle
	SP 10	in vastus medialis muscle, 2 cun superior to upper margin of patella

Meridian	Acupuncture Point	Location
Liver Meridian (LR)	LR 7	1 cun posterior to SP 9
	LR 8	on medial side of knee joint posterior to tibia medial condyle
Kidney Meridian (KI)	KI 10	on medial side of popliteal fossa between semitendinosus and semimembranosus tendons

Extra-Meridian Points

Table 19-2

Point	Location
Knee-Eye	medial to infra-patellar tendon (intra-articular)
Supra-Patellar Tendon point	midpoint superior to upper margin of patella
Infra-Patellar Tendon point	midpoint inferior to lower margin of patella
Ling Hou	inferior and posterior to head of fibula
Baichongwo	1 cun superior to SP 10
Dannang	l cun inferior to GB 34

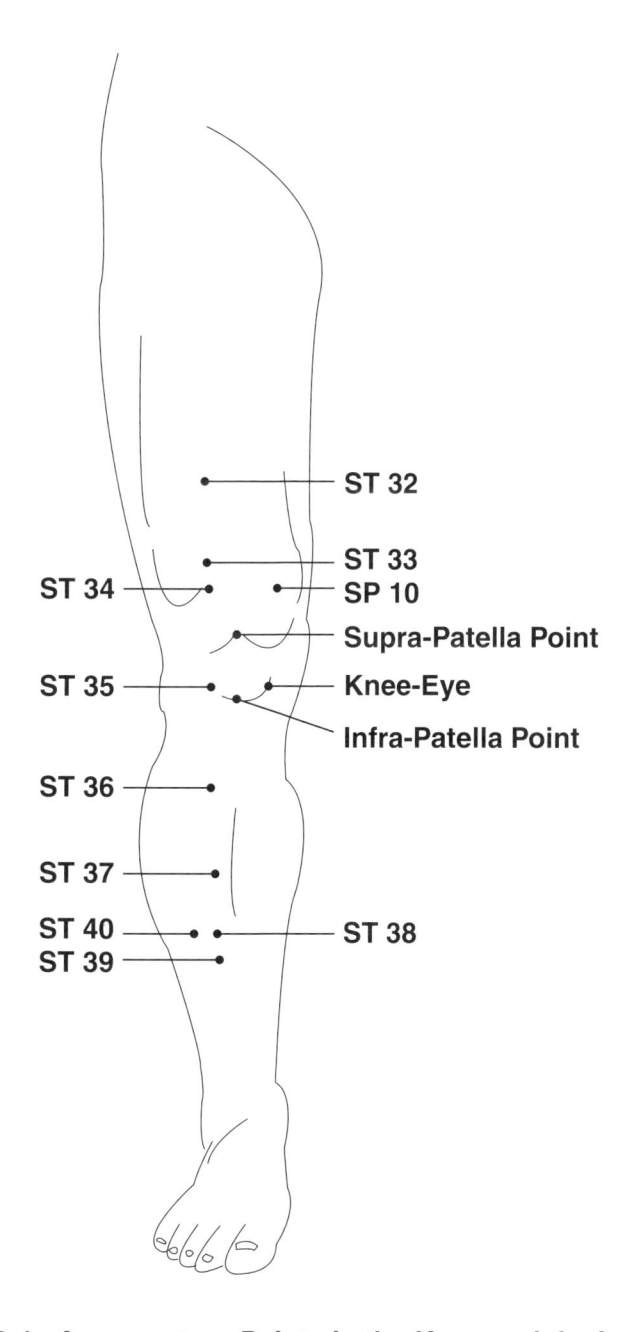

Fig. 19-1. Acupuncture Points in the Knee and the Leg
 - Anterior Surface View

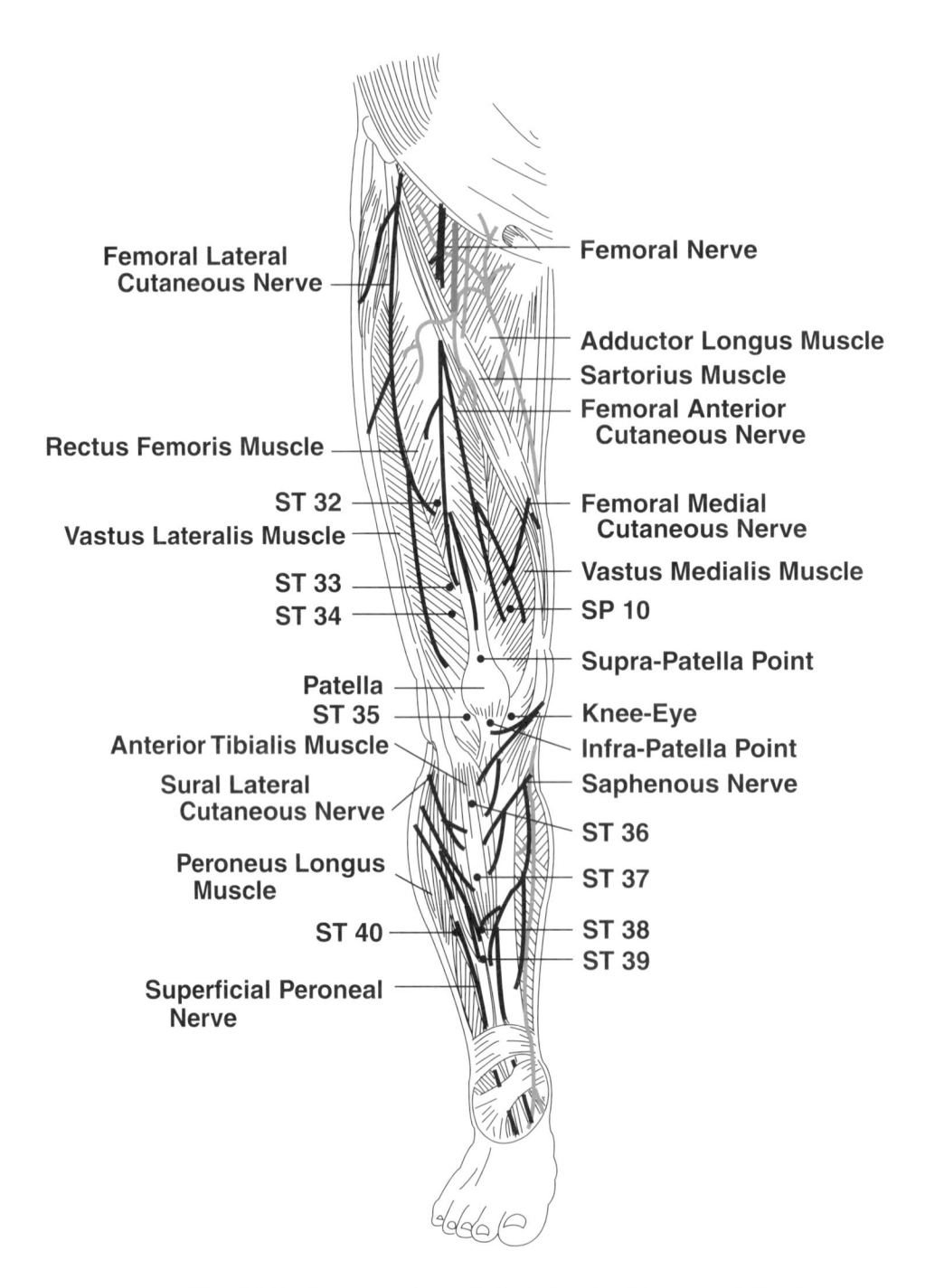

Fig. 19-2. Acupuncture Points in the Knee and the Leg
- Anterior Superficial View

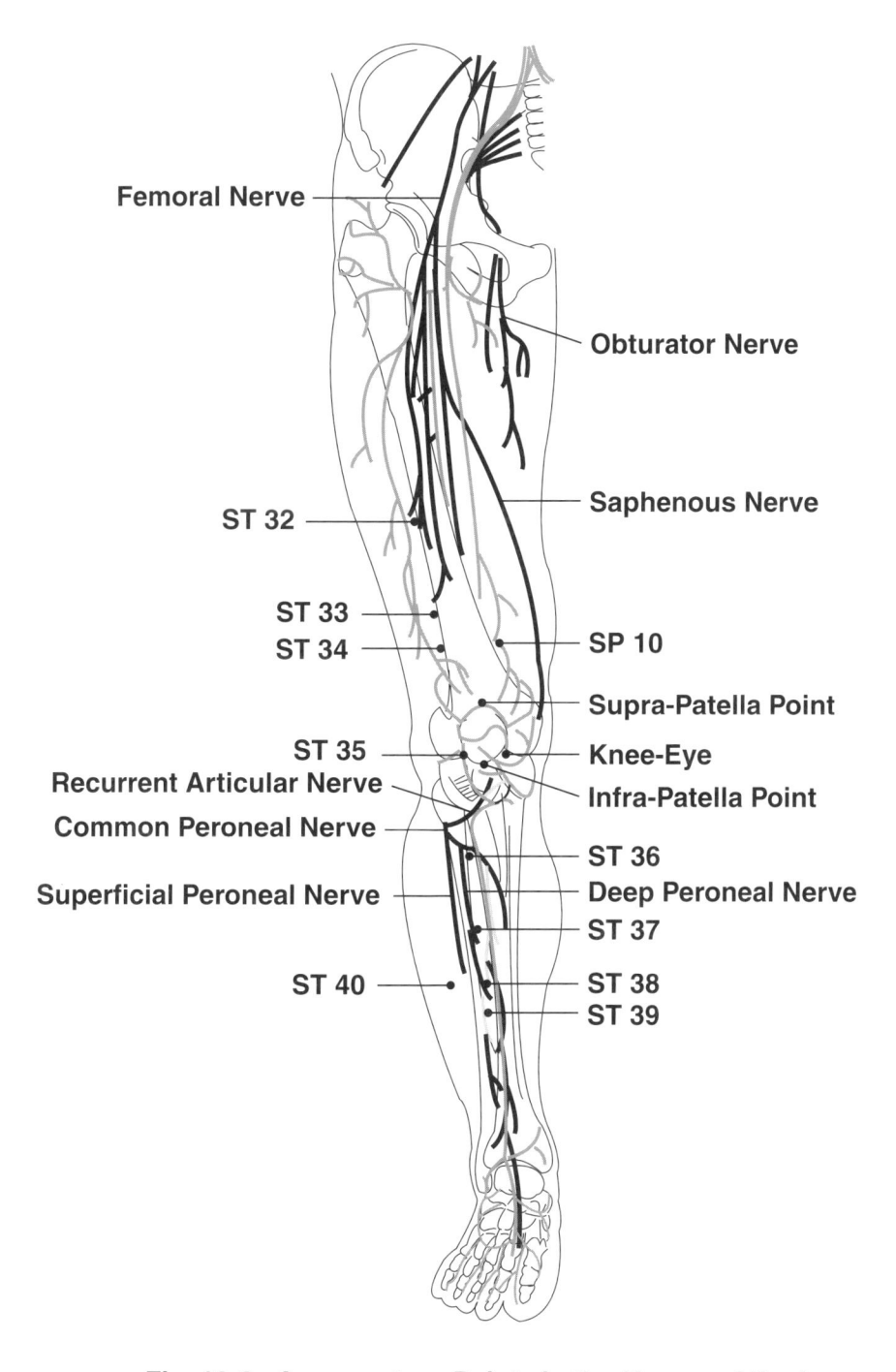

Fig. 19-3. Acupuncture Points in the Knee and the Leg - Anterior Deep View

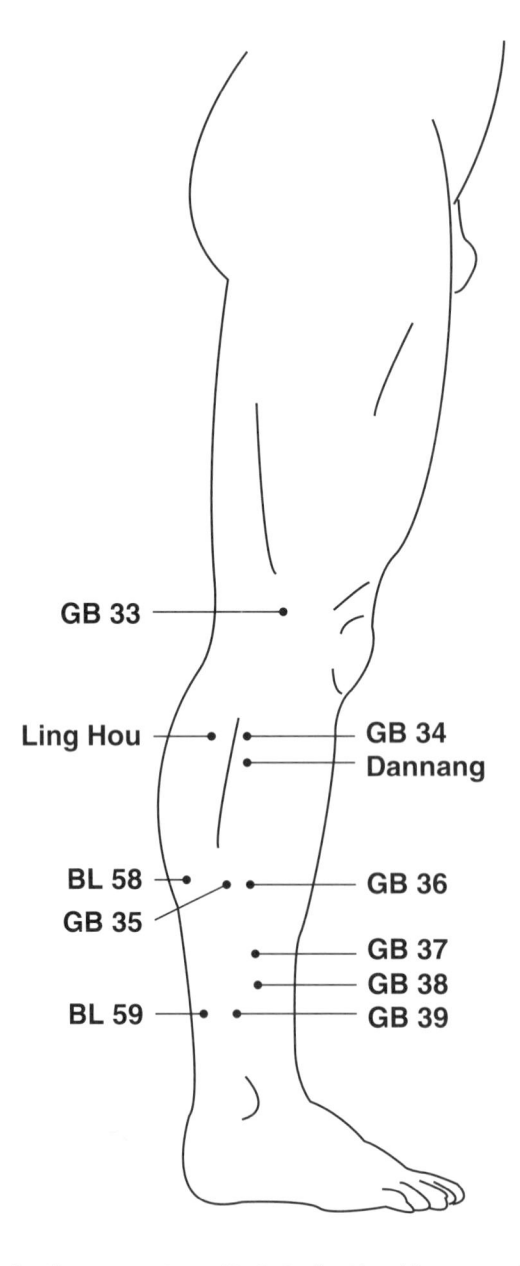

Fig. 19-4. Acupuncture Points in the Knee and the Leg
 - Lateral Surface View

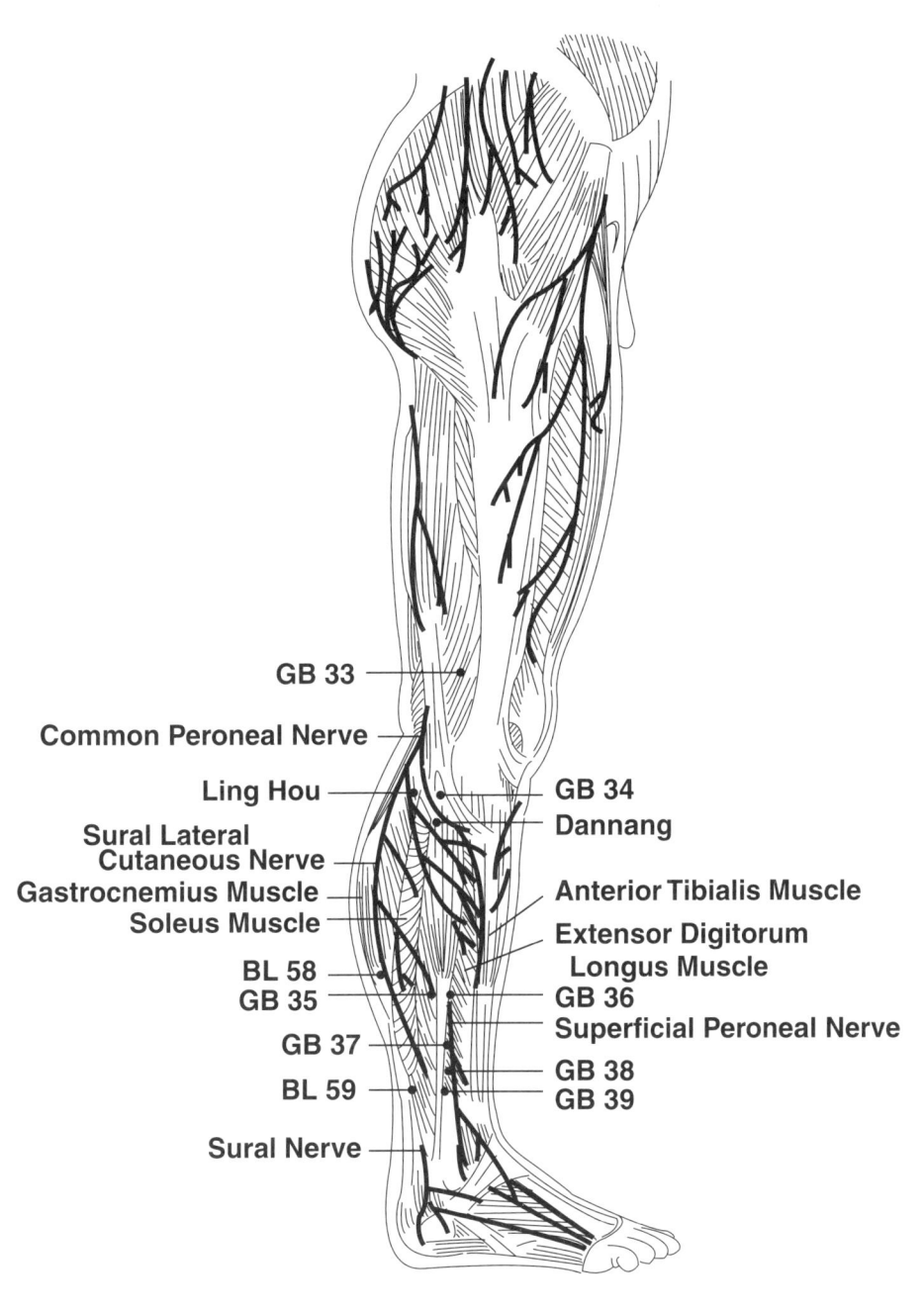

Fig. 19-5. Acupuncture Points in the Knee and the Leg
- Lateral Superficial View

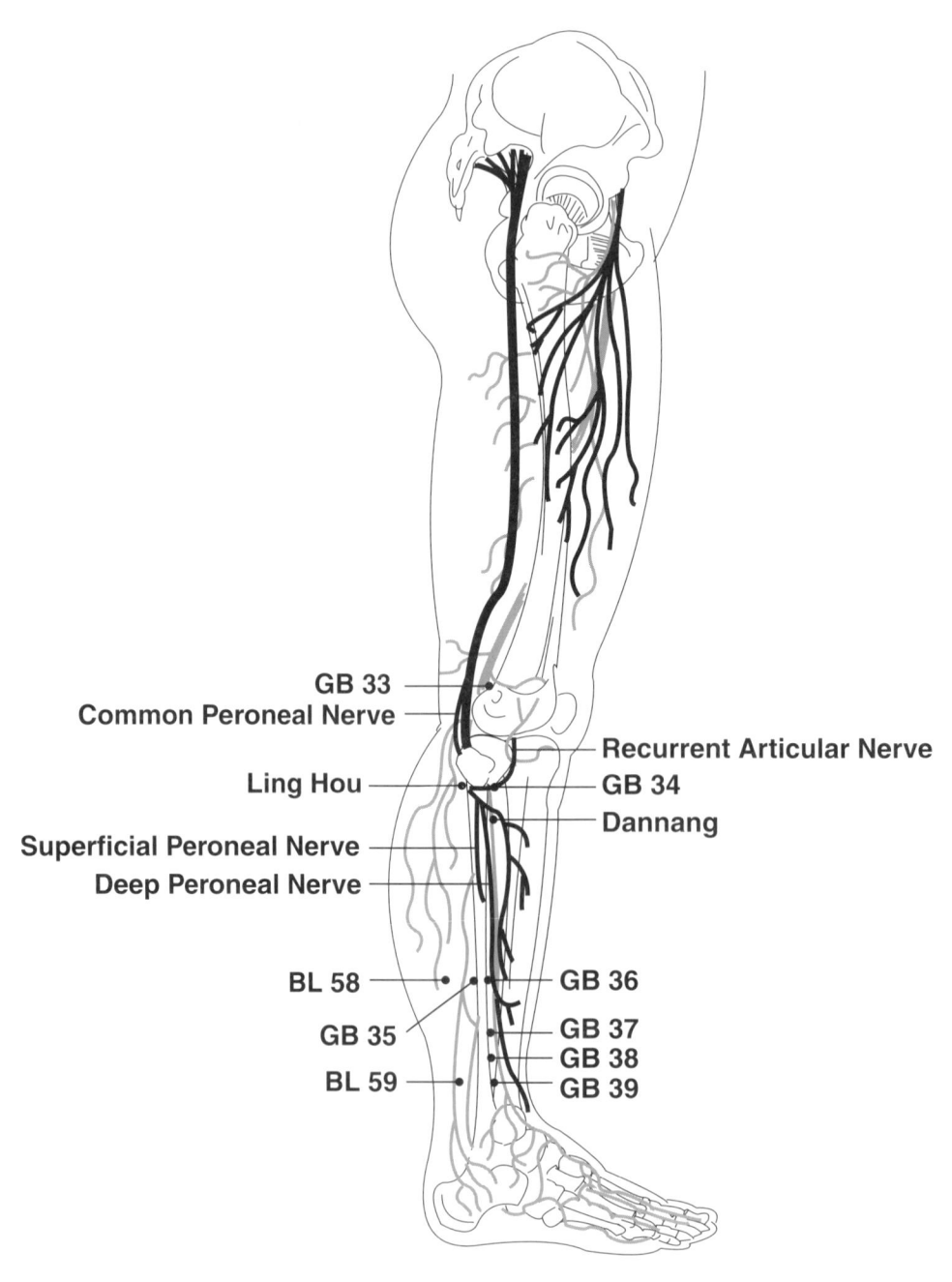

Fig. 19-6. Acupuncture Points in the Knee and the Leg - Lateral Deep View

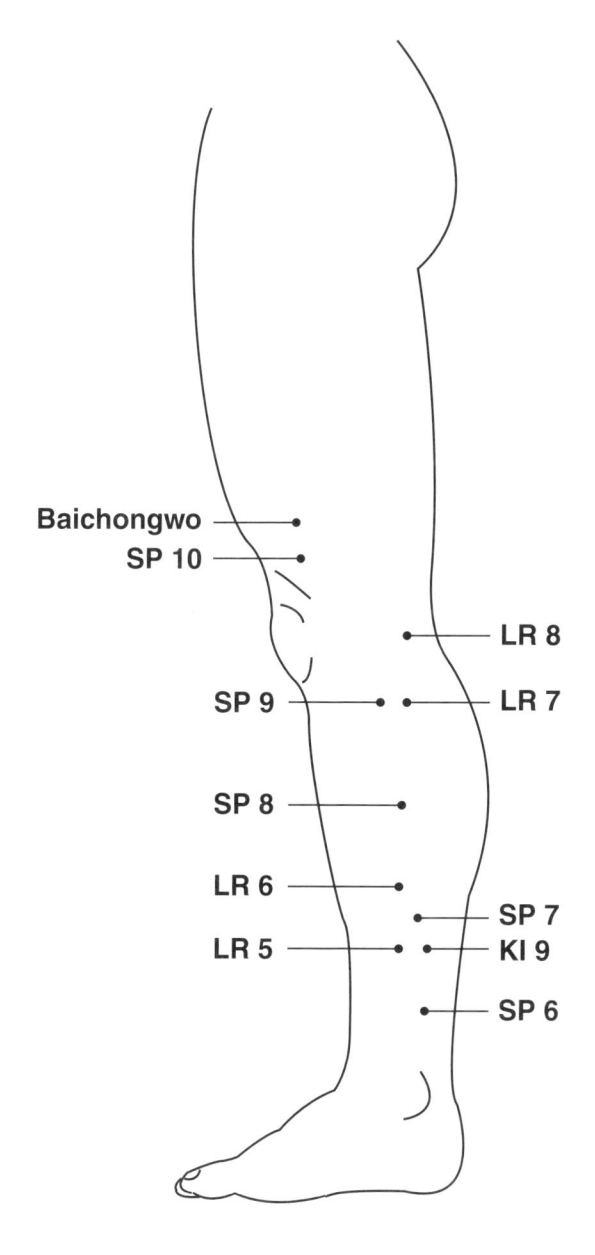

Fig. 19-7. Acupuncture Points in the Knee and the Leg
 - Medial Surface View

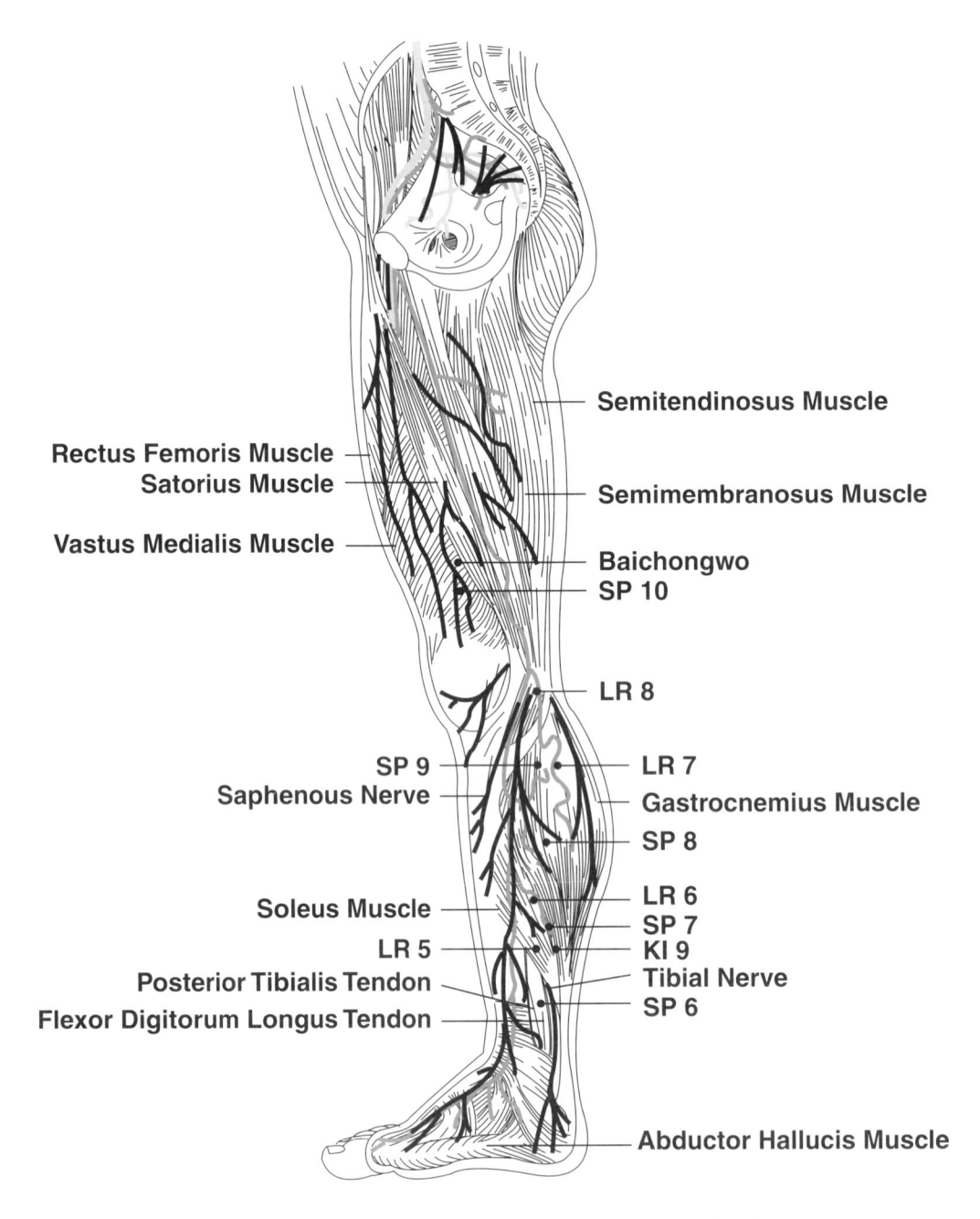

Fig. 19-8. Acupuncture Points in the Knee and the Leg
- Medial Superficial View

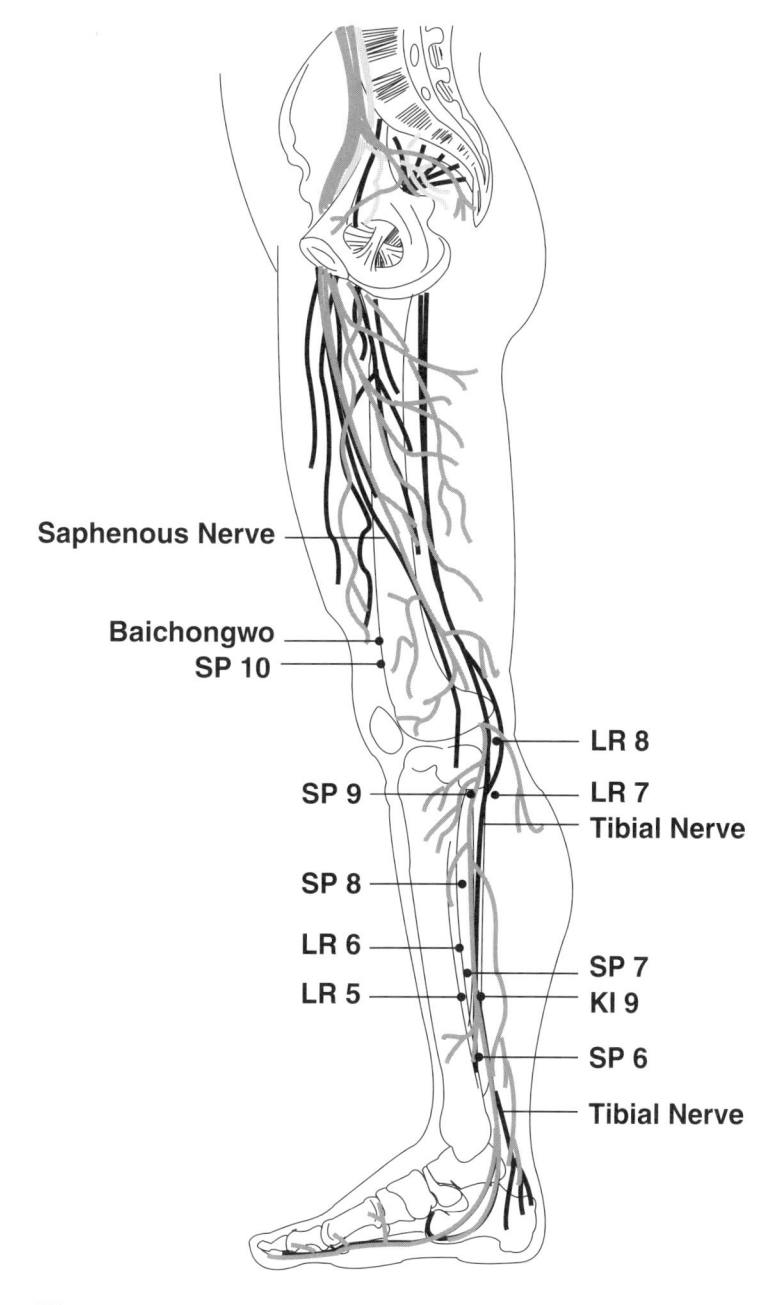

Fig. 19-9. Acupuncture Points in the Knee and the Leg
- Medial Deep View

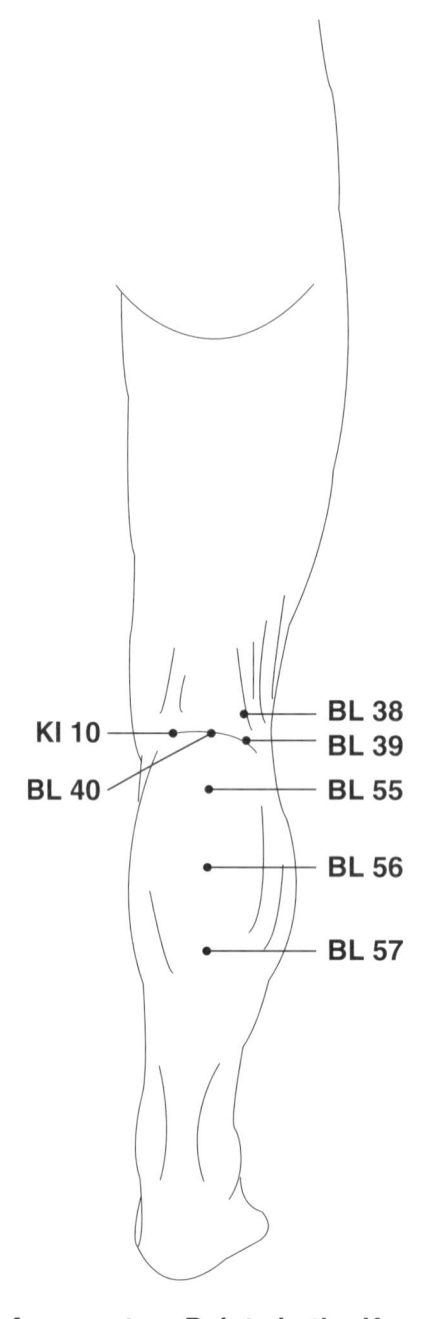

Fig. 19-10. Acupuncture Points in the Knee and the Leg
- Posterior Surface View

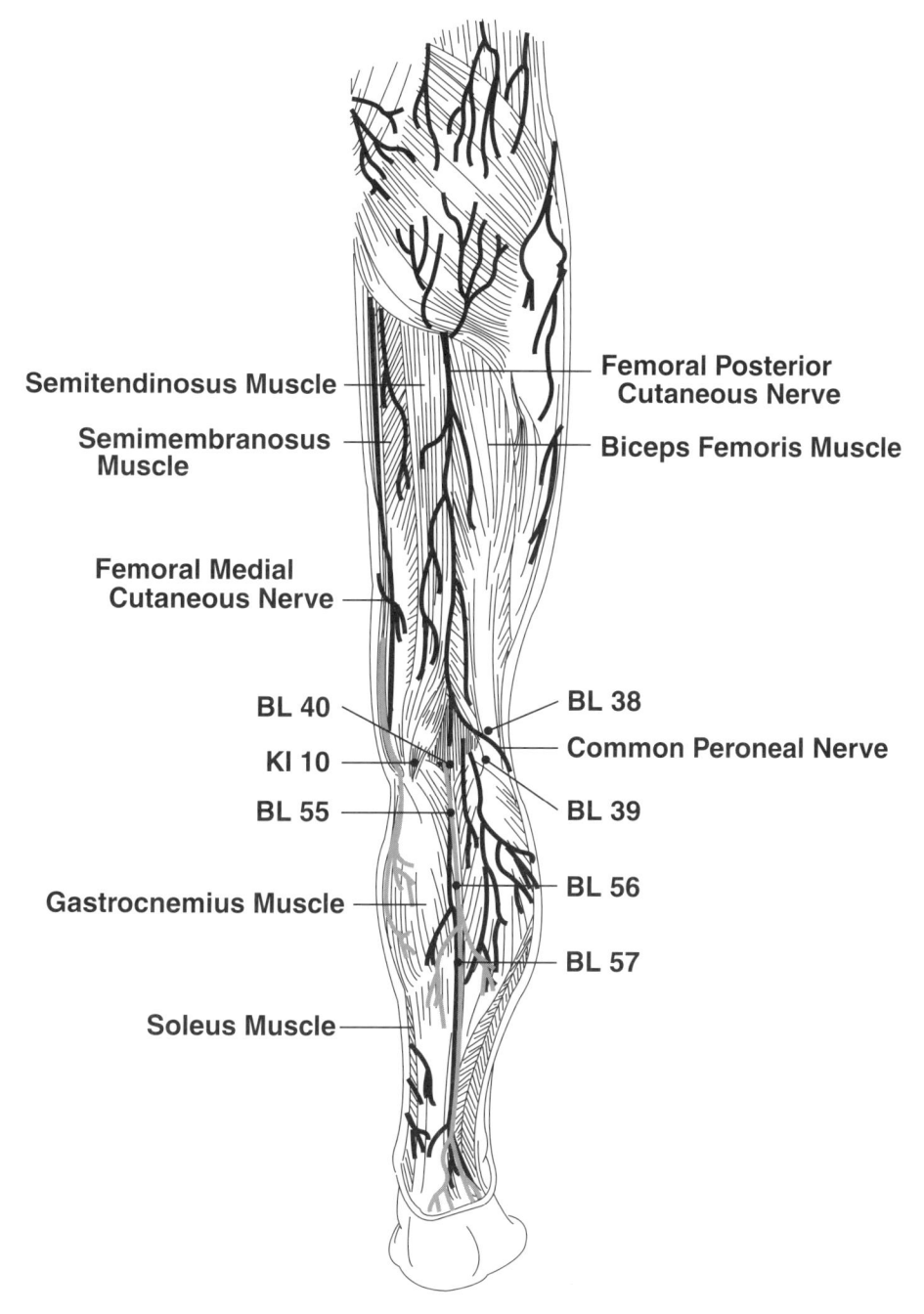

Fig. 19-11. Acupuncture Points in the Knee and the Leg
- Posterior Superficial View

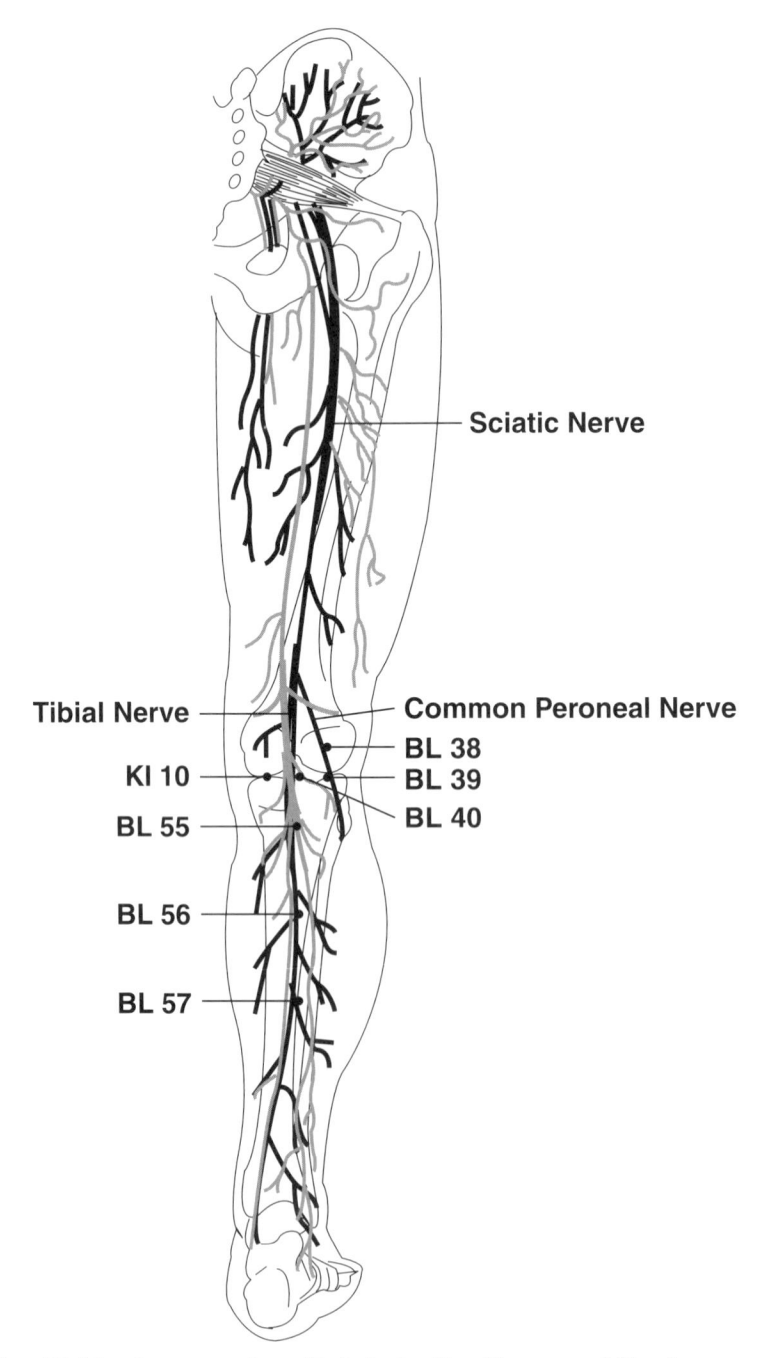

Fig. 19-12. Acupuncture Points in the Knee and the Leg - Posterior Deep View

Nerve Stimulation in the Knee and Leg

Table 19-3

	Name of Nerve	Acupuncture Point
Direct Stimulation to the Knee	knee joint (intra-articular)	ST 35, BL 40, Knee-Eye point, Infra-Patellar point
Peripheral Nerve	femoral nerve	SP 12, ST 32, ST 33, ST 34, SP 10
	peroneal nerve	BL 38, BL 39, GB 34, ST 36, Ling Hou
	tibial nerve	BL 40, SP 9, LR 8

Knee Muscles

Table 19-4

Muscle	Action	Peripheral Nerve	Spinal Segment	Acupuncture Point
Quadriceps Femoris	rectus femoris extends leg,	femoral nerve flexes thigh	L 2 - L 4	SP 12, ST 32
Vastus Medialis	extends leg	femoral nerve	L 2 - L 4	SP 12, SP 10, Baichongwo
Vastus Lateralis	extends leg	femoral nerve	L 2 - L 4	SP 12, ST 34
Vastus	extends leg	femoral nerve	L 2 - L 4	SP 12, ST 32
Sartorius	flexes leg	femoral nerve	L 2, L 3	SP 12
Gracilis	flexes leg	obturator nerve	L 3, L 4	LR 10, LR 11
Biceps Femoris	flexes leg and rotates leg laterally	sciatic nerve	L 5 - S 2	BL 36, BL 37, BL 38, BL 39
Semitendinosus	flexes leg and rotates leg medially	sciatic nerve	L 5 - S 2	BL 36, BL 37, BL 40
Semimembranosus	flexes leg and rotates leg medially	sciatic nerve	L 5 - S 2	BL 36, BL 37, BL 40
Gastrocnemius	flexes leg	tibial nerve	S 1 - S 2	BL 40, BL 55, BL 56, BL 57
Plantaris	flexes leg	tibial nerve	S 1, S 2	SP 6, SP 7, SP 8, SP 9
Popliteus	flexes leg and rotates leg medially	tibial nerve	S 1, S 2	SP 6, SP 7, SP 8, SP 9

Clinical Application

Osteoarthritis or Rheumatoid Arthritis of Knee Joint

- intra-articular points of knee joint: laterally, ST 35; medially, Knee-Eye point; anteriorly, Infra-Patellar point; posteriorly, BL 40

- peripheral nerve stimulation for knee: laterally, GB 34; medially, SP 9; posteriorly, BL 40

- for rheumatoid arthritis, add immune mechanism points: LI 4, ST 36, BL 23, SP 10, SP 6 (see page 106)

Ligamentous Strain

- for lateral collateral ligament: GB 33, GB 34

- for medial collateral ligament: SP 9, LR 8

- for posterior cruciate ligament: ST 35, Infra-Patella point

- for anterior cruciate ligament: Knee-Eye point, Infra-Patellar point

Ilio-Tibial Tract Strain

- ilio-tibial tract inserts into Gerdy's tubercle of tibia

- tensor fascia lata tightens tract and assists extension of knee

- for ilio-tibial tract strain: GB 31, GB 32

- GB 29 stimulates tensor fascia lata

Bursitis

- pre-patellar and infra-patellar bursae commonly involved

- for supra-patellar bursitis: Supra-Patellar point

- for infra-patellar bursitis: Infra-Patellar point

- for pre-patellar bursitis: a combination of above two points

Quadriceps Strain

- for rectus femoris: ST 32
- for vastus medialis: SP 10, Baichongwo
- for vastus lateralis: ST 34
- peripheral nerve stimulation: SP 12 (femoral nerve)

Hamstring Tendinitis

- pain in posterior aspect of knee
- pain reproduced by resisted knee flexion
- for semitendinosus and semimembranosus: LR 8, KI 10, BL 40
- for biceps femoris: BL 38, BL 39, BL 40

Patello-Femoral Syndrome

- inflammation of patella and femoral condyle
- possible abnormal Q angle or deformities – patella alta or patella baja
- abnormal patellar tracking within femoral condylar groove (crepitation on movements)
- for patello-femoral inflammation: Supra-Patellar point, Infra-Patellar point
- for conditioning of quadriceps: SP 10, ST 34, ST 32
- for sympathetic regulation: ST 36

Pes Anserinus Syndrome

- inflammation of hamstrings and pes anserinus bursa
- mimicking medial collateral ligament sprain
- pes anserinus bursitis: SP 8, SP 9
- plantaris tendinitis: SP 9, SP 10
- popliteal tendinitis: SP 8, SP 9

Osgood-Schlatter's Disease

- inflammation of deep infra-patellar tendon bursa
- epiphysitis of anterior proximal tibial epiphysis
- for pain and swelling: ST 36, Infra-Patellar point
- conditioning of quadriceps: ST 34, ST 32, SP 10, Supra-Patellar point

Anterior Compartment Syndrome

- common in runners
- may occur with leg contusion or fractured leg bones
- neurovascular compression: weakness of dorsiflexors and inverters of foot
- for pain and swelling: ST 36, ST 37, ST 38
- for muscle weakness: Ling Hou

Lateral Compartment Syndrome

- common in runners
- may occur with leg contusion or fractured leg bones
- neurovascular compression: weakness of plantar flexors, abductors and evertors of foot
- for pain and swelling: ST 36, ST 40, GB 36, GB 37, GB 38
- for muscle weakness: Ling Hou

Shin Splints Syndrome

- common in sprinters or long distance runners
- localized pain in either posteromedial or anterolateral aspect of leg
- watch for stress fracture of tibia or fibula
- for pain and swelling: SP 6, SP 7, BL 56, BL 57

Chapter Twenty

The Ankle and the Foot

Acupuncture Meridians and Points in the Ankle and the Foot

There are six meridians crossing the ankle and the foot:

Table 20-1

Meridian	Acupuncture Point	Location
Stomach Meridian (ST)	ST 41	on anterior ankle crease, midpoint between extensor digitorum longus and extensor hallucis longus tendons
	ST 42	on cuneiform bone between extensor digitorum longus and extensor hallucis longus tendons
	ST 43	between 2nd and 3rd metatarsal bones
	ST 44	between 2nd and 3rd toes, proximal to margin of web
	ST 45	0.1 cun to lateral corner of 2nd toe's nail
Gall Bladder Meridian (GB)	GB 40	anterior and inferior to lateral malleolus, lateral to extensor digitorum longus tendon
	GB 41	in depression between 4th and 5th metatarsal bones, lateral to extensor digitorum brevis tendon
	GB 42	between 4th and 5th metatarsal bones, 0.5 cun distal to GB 41
	GB 43	between 4th and 5th toes, proximal to margin of web
	GB 44	0.1 cun to lateral corner of 4th toe's nail

Meridian	Acupuncture Point	Location
Urinary Bladder Meridian (BL)	BL 60	in depression between lateral malleolus and Achilles tendon
	BL 61	in depression of lateral surface of calcaneum
	BL 62	in depression inferior to lateral malleolus
	BL 63	in depression on lower border of cuboid bone
	BL 64	inferior to tuberosity of 5th metatarsal bone
	BL 65	inferior to 5th metatarsal bone, proximal to head of 5th metatarsal bone
	BL 66	in depression distal and inferior to 5th metatarsal phalangeal joint
	BL 67	0.1 cun to lateral corner of 5th toe's nail
Spleen Meridian (SP)	SP 1	0.1 cun to medial corner of big toe's nail
	SP 2	on medial side of proximal end of proximal phalanx of big toe
	SP 3	on medial side of distal end of metatarsal bone of big toe
	SP 4	in depression distal and inferior to base of 1st metatarsal bone
	SP 5	in depression distal and inferior to medial malleolus
	SP 6	3 cun superior to tip of medial malleolus on posterior border of tibia
Liver Meridian (LR)	LR 1	0.1 cun to lateral corner of big toe's nail
	LR 2	between 1st and 2nd toes, proximal to margin of web
	LR 3	between 1st and 2nd toes, midpoint at 2nd metatarsal
	LR 4	1 cun anterior to medial malleolus in depression medial to anterior tibialis tendon

Meridian	Acupuncture Point	Location
Kidney Meridian (KI)	KI 1	on sole of foot, between 2nd and 3rd metatarsal bones, proximal to MTT joint
	KI 2	in depression inferior to lower border of tuberosity of navicular bone
	KI 3	in depression between medial malleolus and Achilles tendon
	KI 4	posterior and inferior to KI 3, superior to calcaneus
	KI 5	1 cun inferior to KI 3
	KI 6	in depression inferior to medial malleolus

Extra-Meridian Points

Table 20-2

Point	Location
Bafeng	in webs between toes, eight points in all
Shimian (Insomnia)	at centre of heel
Lineiting	on the planta, in web between 1st and 2nd toes

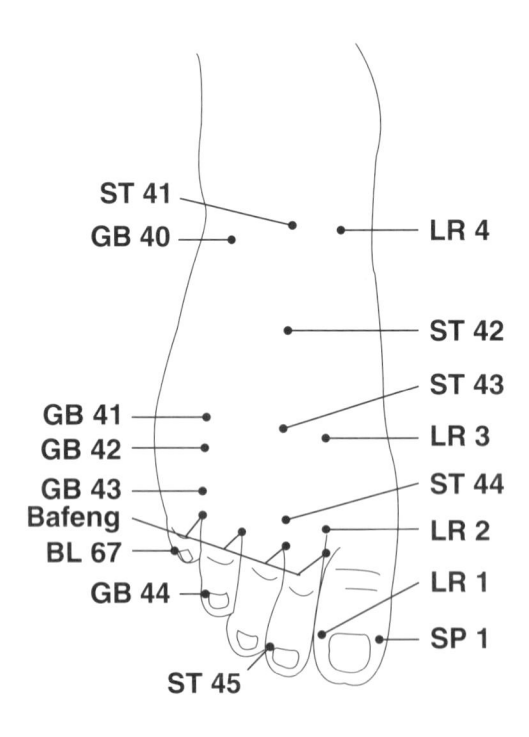

Fig. 20-1. Acupuncture Points in the Ankle and the Foot
- Anterior Surface View

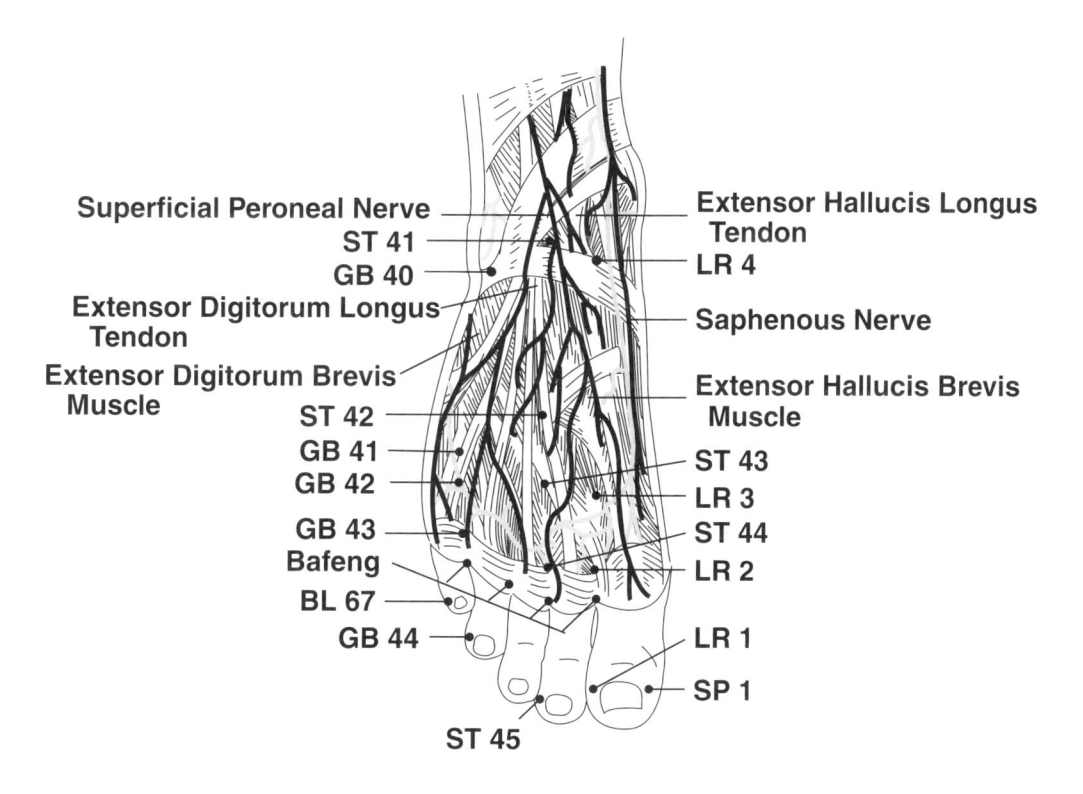

Fig. 20-2. Acupuncture Points in the Ankle and the Foot
- Anterior Superficial View

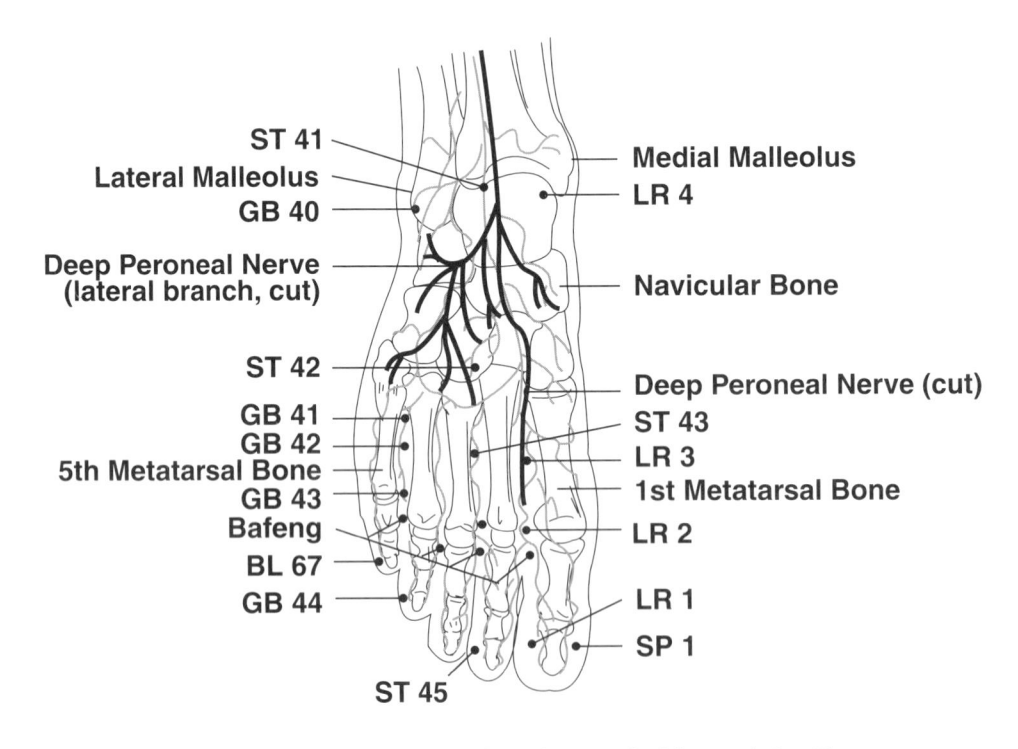

Fig. 20-3. Acupuncture Points in the Ankle and the Foot
- Anterior Deep View

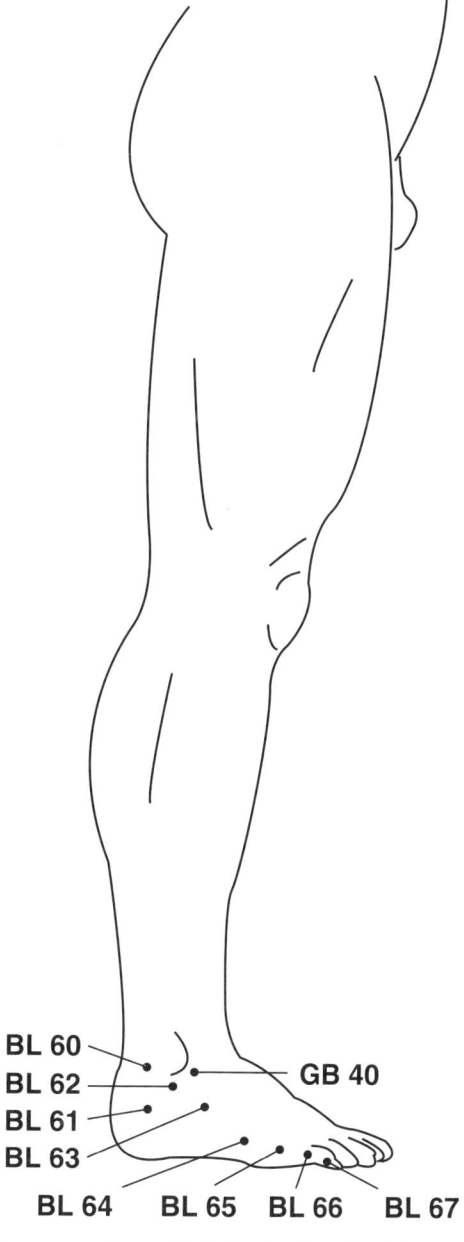

Fig. 20-4. Acupuncture Points in the Ankle and the Foot - Lateral Surface View

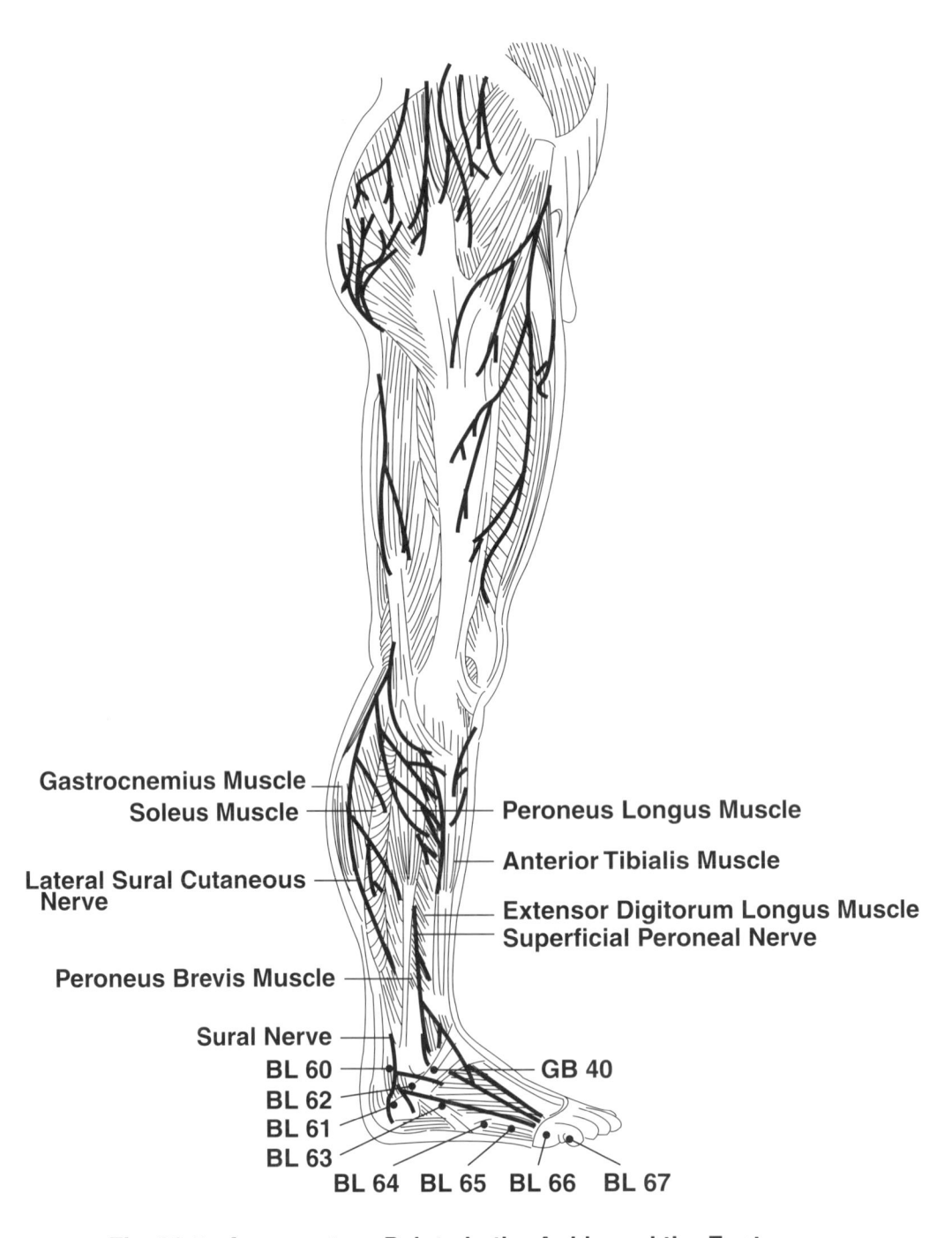

Fig. 20-5. Acupuncture Points in the Ankle and the Foot
- Lateral Superficial View

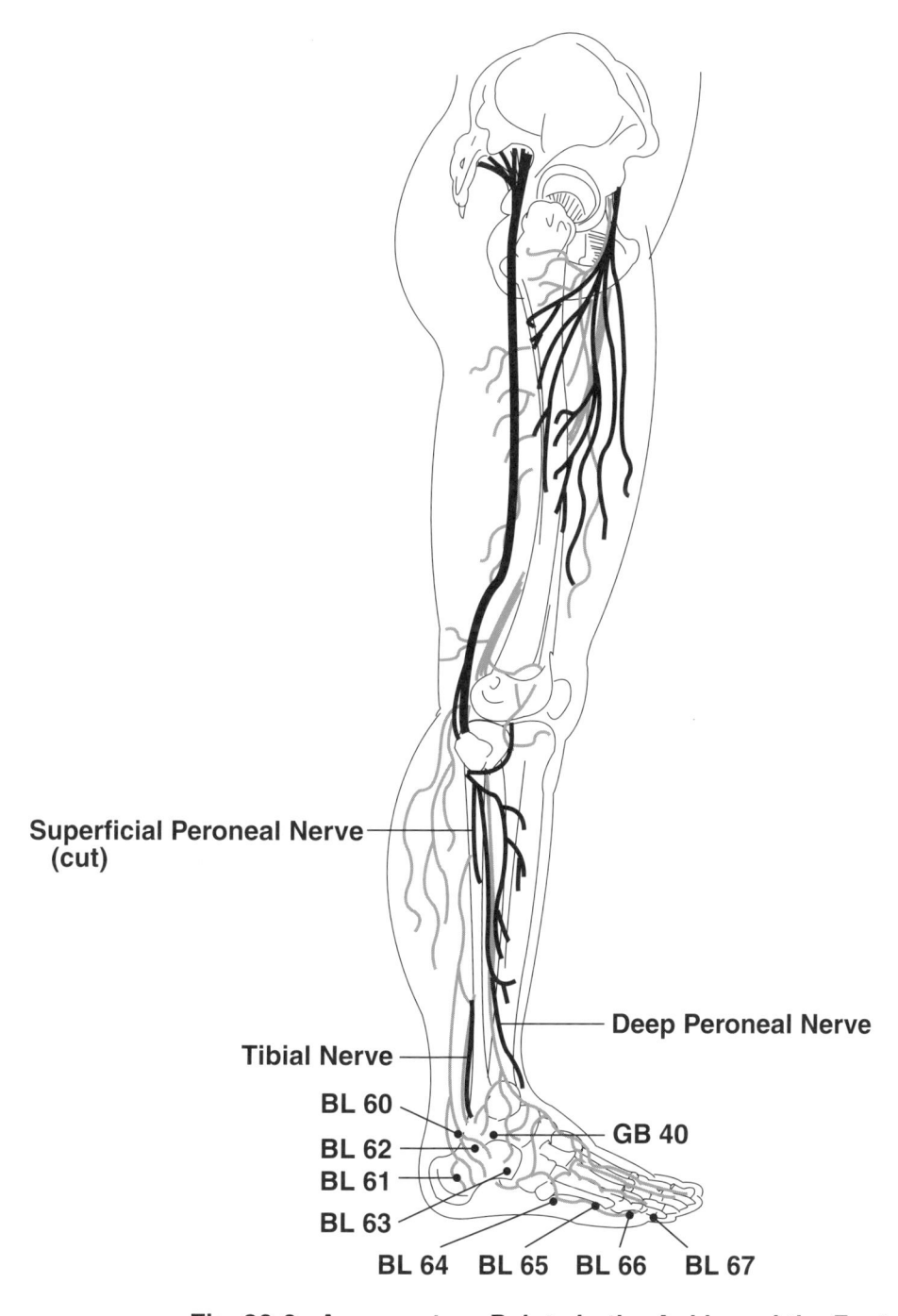

Fig. 20-6. Acupuncture Points in the Ankle and the Foot
- Lateral Deep View

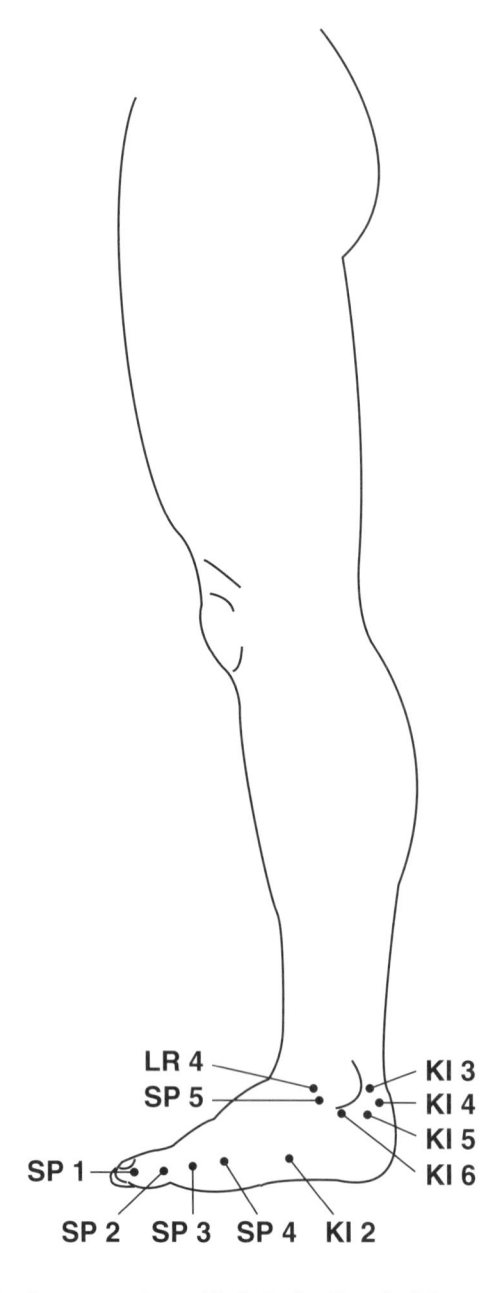

Fig. 20-7. Acupuncture Points in the Ankle and the Foot
- Medial Surface View

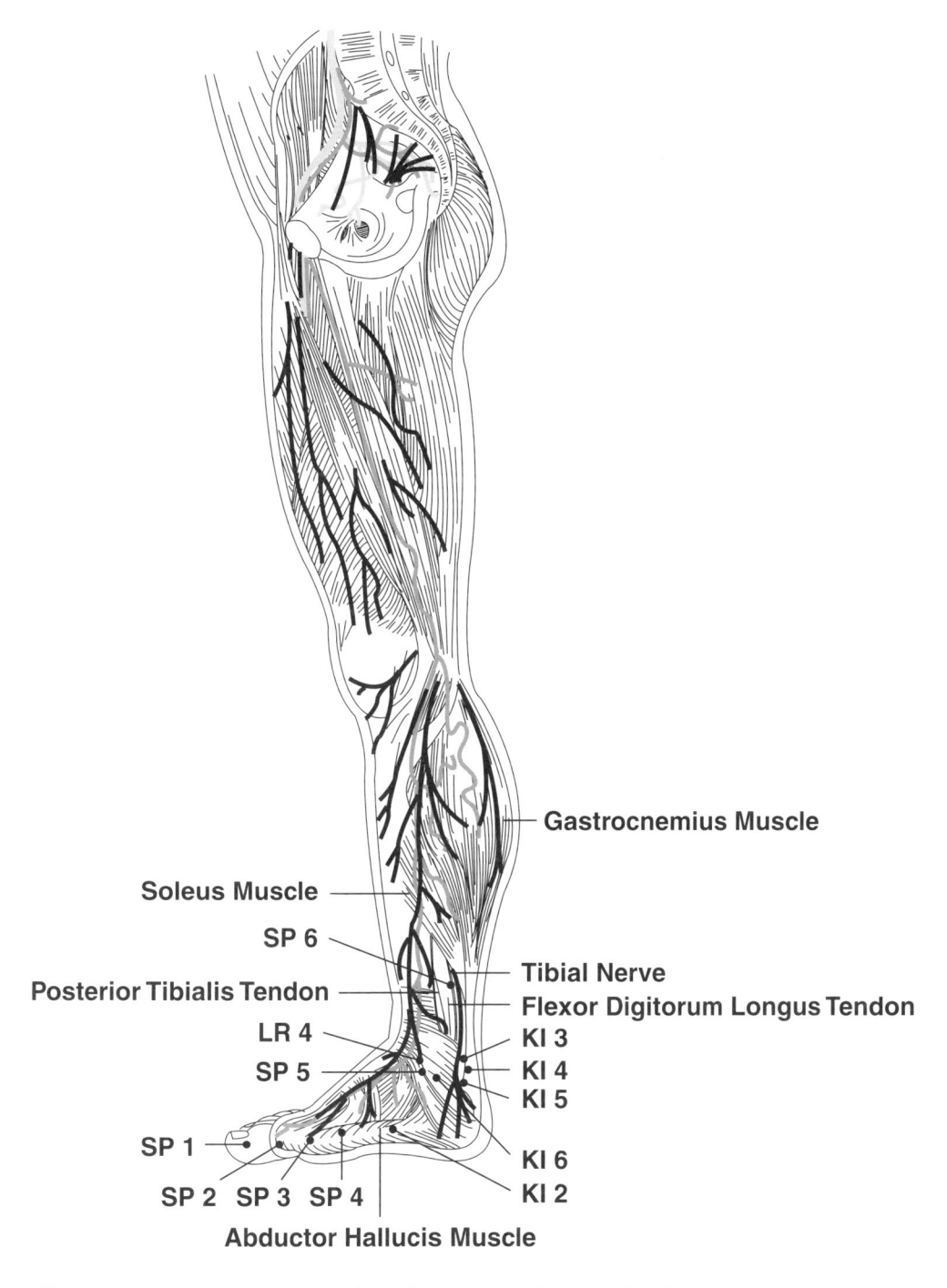

Fig. 20-8. Acupuncture Points in the Ankle and the Foot
 - Medial Superficial View

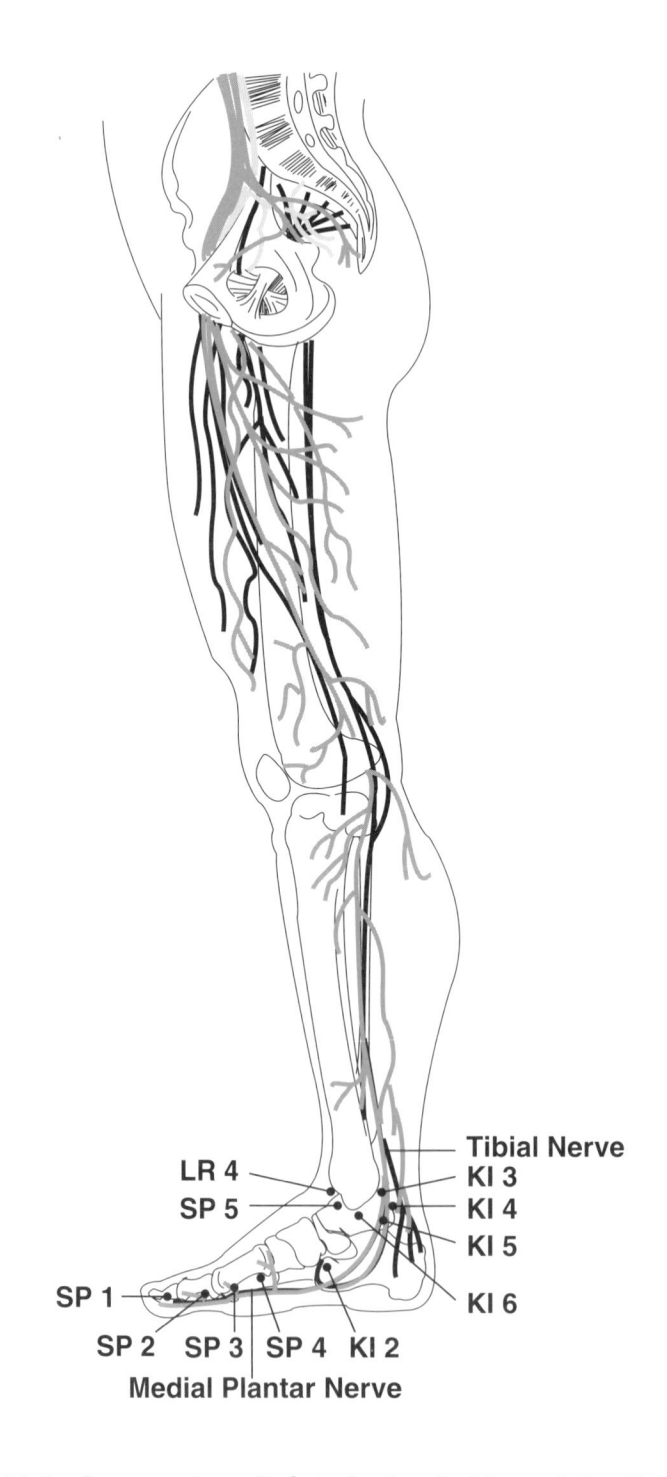

Fig. 20-9. Acupuncture Points in the Ankle and the Foot
- Medial Deep View

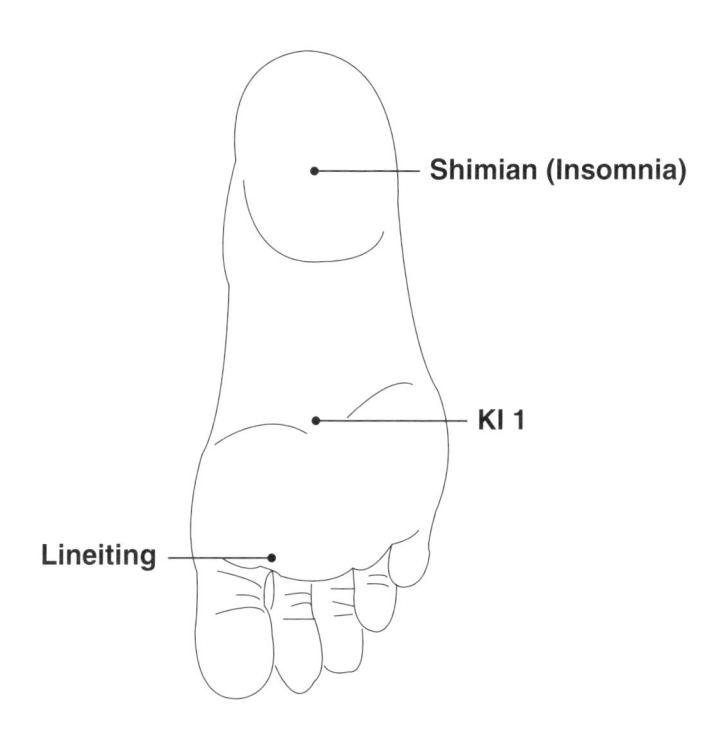

Fig. 20-10. Acupuncture Points in the Foot
 - Plantar Surface View

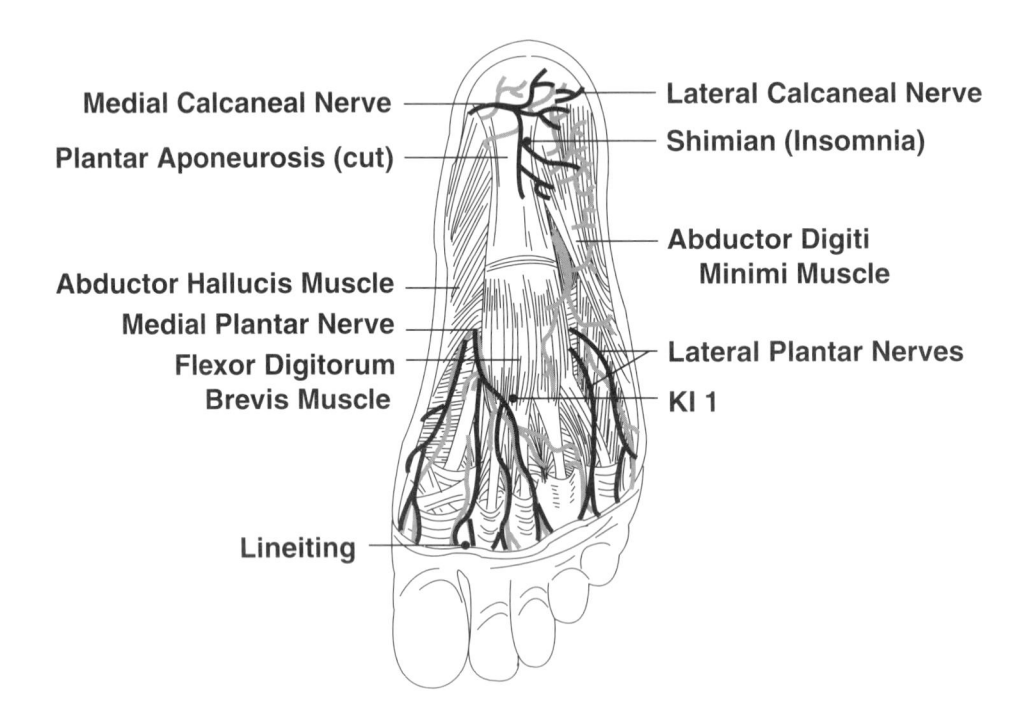

Fig. 20-11. Acupuncture Points in the Foot
- Plantar Superficial View

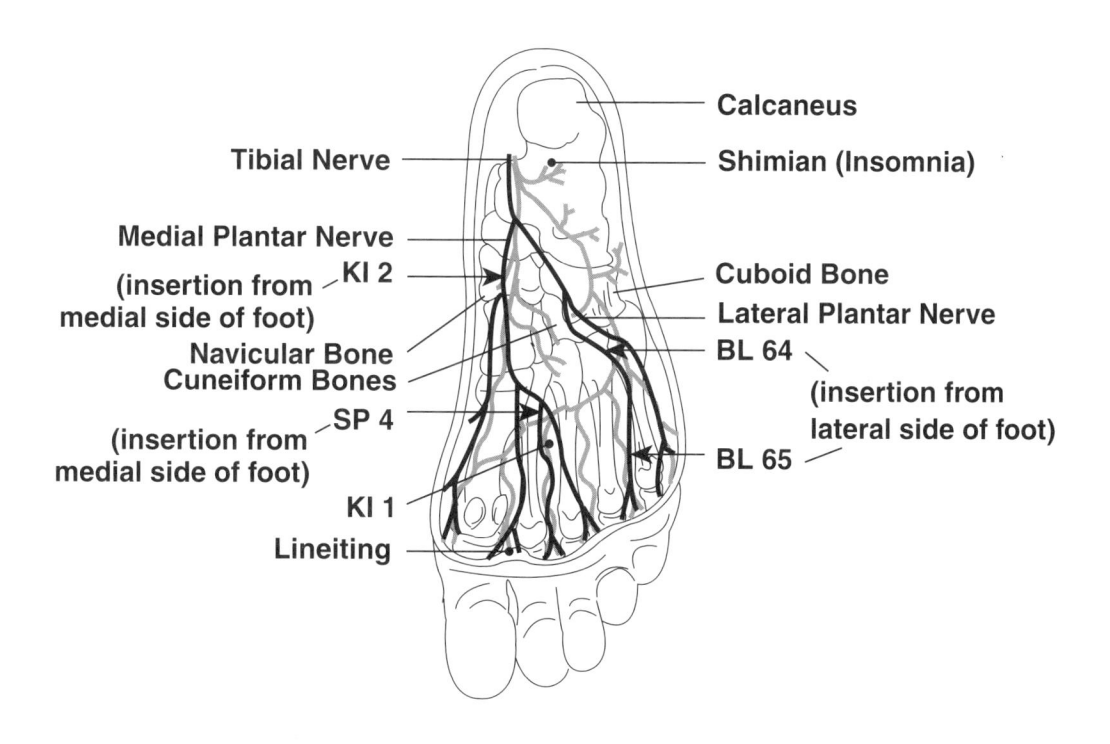

Fig. 20-12. Acupuncture Points in the Foot
- Plantar Deep View

Nerve Stimulation in the Ankle and Foot

Table 20-3

	Name of Nerve	Acupuncture Point
Direct Stimulation to the Ankle	ankle joint (intra-articular)	ST 41
Peripheral Nerve	deep peroneal nerve	ST 41, ST 42, LR 3
	superficial peroneal nerve	GB 40
	sural nerve	BL 60
	saphenous nerve	SP 3, SP 4
	medial plantar nerve	SP 3, SP 4, KI 2
	lateral plantar nerve	BL 64, BL 65, BL 66
	digital nerve	ST 43, ST 44, GB 41, GB 42, GB 43, LR 2, LR 3, Bafeng (eight points in all)

Ankle and Foot Muscles

Table 20-4

Muscle	Action	Innervation Peripheral Nerve	Innervation Spinal Segment	Acupuncture Point
Gastrocnemius	flexes leg, plantar flexes, adducts and inverts foot	tibial nerve	S 1, S 2	BL 56, BL 57, BL 40, SP 8, SP 9
Soleus	plantar flexes, adducts and inverts foot	tibial nerve	S 1, S 2	SP 6, SP 7
Plantaris	flexes leg, plantar flexes foot	tibial nerve	S 1, S 2	SP 6, SP 7, SP 8, SP 9
Flexor Digitorum Longus	flexes digits, plantar flexes and inverts foot	tibial nerve	S 2, S 3	SP 6, KI 3

Muscle	Action	Peripheral Nerve	Spinal Segment	Acupuncture Point
Flexor Hallucis Longus	flexes big toe, plantar flexes and inverts foot	tibial nerve	S 2, S 3	KI 3
Posterior Tibialis	plantar flexes and inverts foot	tibial nerve	L 4, L 5	KI 3, SP 6
Anterior Tibialis	dorsiflexes and inverts foot	deep peroneal nerve	L 4, L 5	ST 36, ST 37
Extensor Digitorum Longus	dorsiflexes foot, everts foot and extends toes	deep peroneal nerve	L 5, S 1	ST 36, ST 37
Extensor Hallucis Longus	extends big toe dorsiflexes foot and inverts sole	deep peroneal nerve	L 5, S 1	ST 39, ST 41
Peroneus Longus	plantar flexes, abducts and everts foot	superficial peroneal nerve	L 5 - S 2	BL 58, BL 59, BL 60, ST 40
Peroneus Brevis	plantar flexes and everts foot	superficial peroneal nerve	L 5 - S 2	BL 59, BL 60, ST 40
Extensor Digitorum Brevis	extends medial four toes	deep peroneal nerve	S 1, S 2	ST 43, ST 44
Flexor Digitorum Brevis	flexes toes	medial plantar nerve	S 2, S 3	SP 4
Abductor Hallucis	abducts big toe	medial plantar nerve	S 2, S 3	SP 4
Flexor Hallucis Brevis	flexes 1st phalanx of big toe	medial plantar nerve	S 2, S 3	SP 4
Adductor Hallucis	adducts big toe	lateral plantar nerve	S 2, S 3	BL 64, BL 65
Abductor Digiti Quinti	abducts and flexes little toe	lateral plantar nerve	S 2, S 3	BL 64, BL 65

Muscle	Action	Peripheral Nerve	Spinal Segment	Acupuncture Point
Flexor Digiti Quinti Brevis	abducts and flexes little toe	lateral plantar nerve	S 2, S 3	BL 64, BL 65
Opponens Digiti Quinti	draws little toe medially and plantarward	lateral plantar nerve	S 2, S 3	BL 64, BL 65
Lumbricales	flexes 1st phalanx	medial plantar nerve	S 2, S 3	Bafeng (eight points in all)
Interossei	abducts and adducts toes	medial plantar nerve, lateral plantar nerve	S 2, S 3	Bafeng (eight points in all)

Clinical Application

Osteoarthritis and Rheumatoid Arthritis in the Ankle

- osteoarthritis uncommon in ankle unless predisposed by previous trauma

- rheumatoid arthritis more common in the smaller joints of foot, add immune mechanism points LI 4, ST 36, BL 23, SP 10, SP 6 (see page 106)

- intra-articular point of ankle: ST 41

- peripheral nerve stimulation for the ankle: medially, KI 3; laterally, BL 60; anteriorly, ST 41

Lateral Collateral Ligament Sprain

- most common ankle injury, commonly due to forced inversion
- grade one – no hemorrhage or clinical instability
- grade two – tearing of ligaments and lateral capsule
- grade three – complete rupture of ligaments and joint capsule
- for grade one and grade two: BL 60, BL 62, GB 40

Medial Collateral Ligament Sprain

- uncommon ankle injury due to forced eversion of foot
- possible tearing of medial ligaments and fracture of medial malleolus
- ankle fracture requires reduction and casting
- acupuncture points: KI 3, KI 6, SP 5

Retrocalcaneal Bursitis

- rectrocalcaneal bursa locating at distal end of Achilles tendon
- "pump bumps" may be co-existing
- painful active dorsiflexion of foot
- acupuncture points: KI 4, in addition to peripheral nerve stimulation: KI 3 (tibial nerve), BL 60 (sural nerve)

Achilles Tendon Strain or Tendinitis

- must rule-out complete tear of tendon
- restrictive taping for partial tears
- acupuncture points: KI 4, BL 57

Plantar Fasciitis

- pain and tenderness under heel
- calcaneal spur may or may not be existing
- possible minor tear of plantar tendon fibres
- possible avulsion of periosteum with subperiosteal inflammation
- acupuncture points: SP 4, BL 61, Lineiting, Shimian

Gouty Arthritis of Foot

- classic site for uric gout involving 1st metatarsal phalangeal joint
- acute attacks and long periods of remission
- during acute attack, LR 2 and LR 3 never fail

Rheumatoid Arthritis and Osteoarthritis in the Foot

- metatarsal phalangeal joints particularly involved
- stiff and painful forefoot – metatarsalgia
- acupuncture points: LR 3, ST 43, GB 42, Bafeng (eight points in all)
- for rheumatoid arthritis, add immune acupuncture points LI 4, ST 36, BL 23, SP 10, SP 6 (see page 106)

Index

A

Acromio-clavicular separation, 148

Acupuncture
    definition of, 29, 45
    foot, 64
    hand, 64
    Korean hand, 64
    neuro-anatomical, 61, 62
    nose, 64
    standard nomenclature, 17-26

Addiction
    control of, 27

American Academy of Medical Acupuncture (AAMA), 1

Analgesia, 27, 31

Ankylosing spondylitis, 130

Anterior compartment syndrome, 225

Anti-inflammation, 27, 31, 33

Auriculo-medicine, 64

B

Blood, 7, 8, 9

Body fluid, 7, 8, 9

Body landmarks, 46

Body units, 46

Brain, 32, 43

Broken needle, 80

Bronze and Iron Ages, 1

Bursitis
    acute sub-deltoid, 148
    gluteal, 203
    ischial, 204
    olecranon, 172
    patella, 223
    psoas, 203
    retrocalcaneal, 245
    trochanteric, 203

C

Carpal tunnel syndrome, 185

Cerebellum, 42, 43, 44

Cerebral cortex, 31, 42

Cervical discogenic paresis or paralysis, 109

Cervical facet syndrome, 106

Cervical sympathetic symptoms, 109

Ching Dynasty, 1

Coccydynia, 133

Complications, 79

Cun, 46-52

D

Degenerative disc disease, 104, 129

de Quervain's tenosynovitis, 185

Dispersing, 58, 59

Disposable needles, 45

E

Electrical stimulation, 56, 57

Electro-acupuncture hazards, 81

Essence, 7

F

Fibromyalgia, 109

Finger measurement, 46, 51

Five elements, 1, 4

Frozen shoulder, 150

Fu-organs, 7

G

Golfer's elbow, 171

Gouty arthritis
    foot, 246

H

Han Dynasty, 1
Hazards, 79
Hemorrhage, 80
Holism, 3
Hypothalamus, 31, 32, 42, 44

I

Immune mechanism points, 106
Immunological response, 30
Infection, 80

L

Lateral compartment syndrome, 225
Lateral epicondylitis, 170

M

Macrocosm, 3
Manual stimulation, 56
Masking of diseases, 81
Medial epicondylitis, 171
Medulla oblongata, 42, 43, 44
Meridians, 11, 13, 14, 15
Microcosm, 3
Mid-brain, 31, 32, 42

N

Needle insertion, 53
Neurotransmitters, 1
Normalization of autonomic nervous dysfunction, 27, 31, 34

O

Occipital neuralgia, 107
Osgood-Schlatter's disease, 225
Osteoarthritis
    ankle, 244
    elbow, 170
    foot, 246
    hand and fingers, 186
    hip, 204
    knee, 223
    neck, 104
    shoulder, 148
    wrist, 185

P

Pain
    acute, 39
    anal, 133
    cervical radicular, 104
    chronic, 40
    control of, 27
    management of, 39, 41
    perineal, 133
Panic switch, 65
Parasympathetic switch, 65, 68
Patello-femoral syndrome, 224
Perforation of viscus, 80
Pes anserinus syndrome, 224
Physical therapy, 27, 29
Physiological negative feedback, 40
Piriformis syndrome, 133
Plantar fascitiis, 246
Pons, 42, 43, 44
Pregnancy, 81
Proportional units, 46, 48, 49, 50

Q

Qi, 7, 8, 9

R

Radial tunnel syndrome, 172

Regeneration, 27, 31, 35

Regenerative response, 30

Rheumatoid arthritis
- ankle, 244
- back, 130
- elbow, 170
- foot, 246
- hand and fingers, 186
- hip, 204
- knee, 223
- neck, 105
- shoulder, 148
- wrist, 185

Rotator cuff syndrome, 149

S

Sacroiliac joint, 115

Scheuermann's disease, 129

Seizure, 79

Shin splints syndrome, 225

Spinal cord, 31, 32

Sprain
- ligamentous (ankle), 245
- sacroiliac, 132

Stone Age, 1

Strain
- Achilles tendon, 245
- hamstring, 204
- hip abductor, 205
- ilio-tibial tract, 223
- intercostal muscle, 129
- ligamentous, 106, 170, 185, 204, 223
- musculo-tendinous, 106, 132, 170
- quadriceps, 205, 224
- rhomboid, 129
- Rider's, 204
- thoraco-lumbar fascia, 132

Sympathetic switch, 65, 68

Syncope, 79

Syndrome differentiation, 3

T

Tendinitis
- Achilles tendon, 245
- bicipital, 149
- hamstring, 224
- lateral epicondyle, 171
- medial epicondyle, 171
- subscapularis, 149

Tennis elbow, 170

Tenosynovitis, 172

Thalamus, 42, 43, 44

Therapeutic ECG, 64

Therapeutic EEG, 64

Therapeutic EMG, 63

Therapeutic strategies, 73-77

Thoracic outlet syndrome, 108

Tonifying, 58, 59

Torticollis, 108

Traditional Chinese Medicine (TCM), 3
- health prevention, 10
- pathology, 9
- treatments, 10

Treatment
- duration of, 58

Trigger finger, 186

V
Visceral manifestation, 7

W
Whiplash injury, 107
World Health Organization (WHO), 18

Y
Yin and Yang, 1, 4
Yuan and Ming Dynasties, 1

Z
Zang-organs, 7